The Multicultural Challenge in Health Education

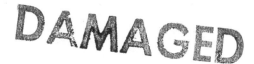

The Multicultural Challenge in Health Education

DAMAGED

Ana Consuelo Matiella, MA, Editor

ETR ASSOCIATES
Santa Cruz, California
1994

ETR Associates (Education, Training and Research) is a nonprofit organization committed to fostering the health, well-being and cultural diversity of individuals, families, schools and communities. The publishing program of ETR Associates provides books and materials that empower young people and adults with the skills to make positive health choices. We invite health professionals to learn more about our high-quality publishing, training and research programs by contacting us at P.O. Box 1830, Santa Cruz, CA 95061-1830, 1-800-321-4407.

Printed in the United States of America
Designed by Ann Smiley
10 9 8 7 6 5 4 3 2 1
Title No. 566

Library of Congress Cataloging-in-Publication Data

The Multicultural challenge in health education / Ana Consuelo Matiella.
    p. cm.
    Includes bibliographical references.
    ISBN 1-56071-355-0
    1. Health education—United States. 2. Minority students—Education (Secondary)—United States.
    I. Matiella, Ana Consuelo.
    RA440.3.U5M85 1994
    610'.71'273—dc20   93-44541

Contents

DAMAGED

Comprehensive Health Education in a Multicultural World

Multicultural Relevancy in Instruction

Increasing Staff Capabilities

Working Together: Family and Community Involvement

Appendix

Preface

Healthy People, published in 1978, laid the foundation for this nation's efforts to pursue a policy of disease prevention and health promotion as a means for improving the health of our citizens. The subsequent publications, *Health Promotion, Disease Prevention: Objectives for the Year 1990,* and *Healthy People 2000: National Health Promotion and Disease Prevention Objectives* identified goals, established target objectives and set forth strategies for improving the health of Americans. One overall important goal established in the year 2000 health objectives was "To reduce (health status) disparities among Americans."

America has been called "The Land of Opportunity." Immigrants from around the world come here seeking a better life for themselves and their children. Religious freedom, economic opportunity, political refuge and better quality of life are all dreams this great nation of ours has, signifying hope for millions of people. With these dreams comes the expectation that education will be the key that opens the door to these opportunities. Hard-earned tax dollars will be used to provide our children with quality education that will prepare them for the future.

However, the health status of all citizens is not equal. America's poor, and especially our children and youth, experience substandard health, and poverty and subsequent poor health are more common in families of color. Although ethnic and cultural diversity is not new to us, America is entering an era in which diversity is even more in the forefront. Historically, education has been designed by the dominant society. Today, we recognize that if the needs of our multiculturally diverse student population are to be met, educational approaches need to change and become more inclusive. We need to open our hearts and our minds to a culturally diverse approach to education and allow our diversity to be our strength. American education needs to build on the strengths of the many cultures represented in our people.

Our nation's educational system is in a state of change. We are on the threshold of great opportunity. Our children are the future of America and the world. One of the United States' greatest opportunities is to succeed in the education of all children. A key to that success is approaching education from a multicultural perspective.

Helping young people acquire the knowledge and skills to practice healthy lifestyles will enable them to prepare themselves for the future. Understanding different cultural needs and values is critical in the process of preparing young people to make healthy choices. It is imperative that educators build on the strengths of cultural values and family beliefs when designing health education programs. Comprehensive school health programs can serve as a unifying force for multicultural education.

The *Multicultural Challenge in Health Education*, written by leading authorities, is a collection of chapters outlining strategies for making health education culturally relevant. The content of these chapters ranges from defining culturally relevant health education to identifying strategies useful in designing and implementing educational programs that build on the strength of America's richly diverse student population.

The goal of this book is to challenge teachers, school administrators, policy-makers and community members to work together to improve the quality of health education, making it relevant to all students. I have faith that we can meet that challenge.

A Word About Ethnic Terms

The current descriptors for racial and ethnic groups vary across the United States by different regions, communities and national identification. In deference to the nomenclature used by the authors and those in use among the various communities, racial and ethnic groups will be identified throughout the book by the various terms used by the authors.

---

*Foundations
for Multicultural
Health Education*

Chapter 1

Who Are the Children and How Is Their Health?

Iris M. Tropp and Marie J. Montrose

Youth under 18 years of age constitute approximately 26 percent of the entire American population, with the proportion of minorities in this age bracket continuing to climb. In 1980, minorities accounted for 26 percent of all youth under age 18. A decade later, this percentage had increased to 31 percent. This trend is apparent across all minority categories, although it is most dramatic for Asian Americans and Hispanics. A summary of these trends is provided in Figure 1. Even though African-American youth are still in the majority, their proportion relative to other minorities has declined from 56.2 percent to 48.4 percent since 1980. Hispanics now comprise 39.2 percent of the minority youth population, followed by Asian Americans who now account for one-tenth of minority youth (Center for the Study of Social Policy, 1992).

Figure 1
Proportion of American Youth
Who are Minorities, 1980–1990

	1980	1990
% U.S. population under 18	28.1	25.6
% Minority population under 18	26.2	31.1
Whites under 18	78.6	74.9
African Americans under 18	14.7	15.1
Hispanics under 18	8.8	12.2
Asian Americans under 18	1.6	3.3
Native Americans under 18	0.9	1.1
Other minorities under 18	4.2	5.7

Source: Kids Count Data Book: State Profiles of Child Well-Being. 1992. Center for the Study of Social Policy, Washington, DC.

When defining the health status of minority youth, the broadest definition of health must be applied, including indicators of social and economic well-being. Inherent in this discussion is the question of which issues, problems and concerns can successfully be addressed through institutions that serve these youth, in particular the public schools. Health status and learning are inextricably linked. Students with untreated health problems may perform poorly in school. Children who are malnourished or have mild deficiencies may have decreased attention spans, be more irritable, or lose concentration easily. Neglect, domestic violence, and emotional trauma can encourage aggressive, disruptive, withdrawn, or depressed behavior and increase stress-induced health concerns (Kolbe, 1985; National Education Association, 1989).

Because comprehensive school health programs are based on the premise that providing information and services which alter behavior will improve the health of children and adults, its core will ultimately be focused on the development of personal awareness and responsibility. This chapter will illustrate that although much of the physical and mental harm incurred by school-age youth results from events which extend beyond the traditional school setting, it can be minimized by effective delivery of school-based health-promotion programs.

Public schools are microcosms of their surrounding communities, reflecting both their social and economic levels. With many middle and upper middle class families diverting their children to private schools, public schools currently enroll a disproportionate number of children from less privileged households. To many professionals working in public schools, this constitutes an additional burden on an already overtaxed system. While this may be true to some degree, it also provides public schools with a window into the future. Schools have far greater potential than other institutions to recognize and address behaviors that could lead to diminished health. Consistent access to youth allows for the early identification of and intervention for health-compromising behaviors. In essence, the public school system is an ideal arena for designing innovative and adaptable strategies for health promotion which reflect the cultural and social needs of minority and low-income populations. Public schools are in a prime position to lead other local, state and national organizations toward improving the health of youth.

Public schools today, especially in large urban areas, represent both minority and low-income groups. Therefore, the following presentation and discussion of statistics and trends must consider economic, social and cultural factors. A common result from demographic studies of minorities in the United States is that economic stability more than racial or ethnic identification is solidly correlated with health knowledge, access to health services, and, ultimately, health status. The proportion of American children living in poverty continues to grow. Minorities fare worse economically than other segments of society, with incomes considerably below the national average (Center for the Study of Social Policy, 1992). As will be shown, a substantial percentage of these fast-growing ethnic groups live below the poverty level and consequently suffer from socially related health problems.

As one ponders "How is their health?", the data must be analyzed with additional questions in mind. For example, are health education and services simply unavailable to these groups? Are economic factors alone responsible for observed declines in health status? Are there cultural habits which prevent or inhibit the utilization of existing service and information channels? Whatever the questions, the answers must be articulated for the benefit of those communities affected, and for the use of those community leaders responsible for providing appropriate health information and services.

The Socioeconomic Picture

Over one-half of the African-American, Hispanic, Native-American, and Asian children in the United States live in poverty. It is estimated that within the next decade, 15 percent of students in public school will be immigrants who do not speak English. These youth are at greater risk for dropping out of school and subsequently have higher unemployment rates as adolescents and adults (Resnick and Hibbard, 1988). After the year 2000, it is estimated that one-third of Americans will be people of color. Their rates of adolescent pregnancy, sexually transmitted disease (STD), substance use, unintentional injury and homicide are substantially higher than the national average (U.S. Census Bureau, 1990). Nationally, one-fifth of teenagers have some sort of illness, deformity or handicap; the rates are much higher in several minority subgroups. One study of inner-city youth found that over half of this population had health-related problems that required intervention (National Center for Health Statistics, 1973).

There are striking differences between minority groups. For example, African-American and Hispanic median incomes average $19,000 to $22,000, compared with a national average of $34,000. In fact, African Americans, Hispanics and Native Americans have below-average median incomes and educational levels, accompanied by higher unemployment rates. Although the average American family's income has decreased by approximately 5 percent in the last decade, African-American and Hispanic households have experienced more dramatic losses. Hispanic family earnings in particular, declined over 11 percent during this same time period (Center for the Study of Social Policy, 1992).

In 1990, the U.S. poverty threshold was established at $13,360 for a family of four with one parent. Forty-five percent of African-American children and 41 percent of Hispanic children under 16 years of age live below the poverty level. Poverty among Hispanics, in particular, seems to be strongly associated with country of origin. On average, Puerto Rican families have lower incomes than Mexican Americans, while Cuban American families exhibit higher income levels than other Hispanic groups (Dryfoos, 1990). Relative to other minorities, Asian Americans have a higher median income and average level of education. However, there is some evidence to suggest that the socioeconomic status of Asian Americans is also closely linked to the country of birth, duration of residence in the United States, and degree of acculturation (Lin-Fu, 1988).

Mortality Data and Health Status

According to a report by the Secretary's Task Force on Black and Minority Health, all of the six leading causes of death for minorities—cardiovascular and cerebrovascular diseases; cancer; chemical dependencies; diabetes; homicide, suicide and unintentional injuries; and infant mortality and low birth weight—have preventable risk factors (U.S. Department of Health and Human Services, 1985). Smoking, alcohol abuse, poor diet, and stress are among the salient risk factors associated with these leading causes of death. It is widely believed that proper education and availability and use of preventive services would substantially reduce excessive deaths among minorities. By providing an overview of the current and projected demographic trends, this chapter attempts to summarize the current health status and future health needs of four minority groups: African Americans, Asian Americans, Hispanics and Native Americans. The data presented emphasize some national trends and are by no means comprehensive. They are meant to shed light on health states and behaviors that are primarily preventable and provide a foundation from which to further explore health and welfare issues for culturally diverse populations. Data are reported for each of these groups whenever possible and appropriate.

For the purposes of interpreting data from a variety of sources, the following general definitions were applied to each group: African American refers to individuals who identify themselves as racially Black, and who may originate from any country (including the Caribbean); Asian American is used to describe anyone of Asian descent, namely Chinese, Filipino, Japanese, East Indian, Korean, Vietnamese, and people from other countries in the Pacific Rim; Hispanic refers to individuals who originate from Spanish-speaking countries, including Mexico, Puerto Rico, Cuba, Spain, Central America and South America; Native American encompasses individuals most commonly referred to as American Indians and Alaska Natives. As is evident from these descriptions, the basis of these four divisions is somewhat arbitrary and leaves statistical information vulnerable to oversimplification, generalization, misinterpretation and possible misapplication. Again, this information is provided only as a very general guide to discovering the complex diversity of multiethnic communities and the ensuing difficulties in fulfilling their multifaceted needs.

In general, minority populations tend to have higher birth rates. Native Americans seem to have the highest birth rates, followed by Hispanics (particularly Mexican Americans and Puerto Ricans), and then African Americans. On average, larger proportions of African Americans, Hispanics and Native Americans are in younger age brackets. One striking example is that over half of the Native-American population is between 0 and 24 years of age (U.S. Department of Health and Human Services, 1992). As age-adjusted mortality rates illustrate, this trend toward a younger population probably reflects early deaths in addition to higher birth rates.

Dramatic decreases in age-adjusted mortality rates for minorities in the United States have occurred during the last few decades. This can be quite deceptive, however. Although the differences between minority and majority rates have lessened, the age-adjusted mortality rate for African Americans is still over 50 percent higher than that of the general population. This rate reflects a higher incidence of heart disease, stroke and cancer, as well as homicide, which is six times higher for African Americans. Native Americans have virtually the same mortality rates as the general population and exhibit lower death rates for most chronic diseases. However, they do show much higher rates for death at earlier ages from accidental injuries (especially motor vehicle) and chronic liver disease which are strongly related to the prevalence of alcohol consumption and uncontrolled diabetes (U.S. Department of Health and Human Services, 1992).

Behaviors that cause most adolescent deaths are influenced by social factors and are preventable. The leading causes of teen deaths in the United States are accidents (mostly motorcycle and automobile), suicide and homicide, followed by cancer, heart disease and chronic conditions (Schaffer et al., 1987). Violent deaths among older teens, ages 15 to 19, are increasing steadily. By the end of the 1980s, over two-thirds of the states in the nation reported increases in teen deaths due to homicide, suicide and accidents, with the entire country experiencing an 11 percent increase overall. A 62 percent increase in violent deaths among Hispanic teens alone was noted in the past decade (Center for the Study of Social Policy, 1992).

African-American and Native-American youth ages 0 to 14 are also much more likely to die from intentional and unintentional injuries than the rest of the population. African-American youth are three and one-half times as likely to perish as a result of homicide, while Native-American youth are twice as likely as majority youth. Similar rates are found for deaths by household fires. Native-American youth are also twice as likely to die by suicide or in motor vehicle crashes (Waller, Baker and Szocka, 1989). Deaths of this sort, by homicide, suicide, fire and car crashes, most likely reflect the poor living conditions and unsafe communities these youth are exposed to as a result of the less stable economic and educational base of their parents. In addition to the fatalities associated with violence, minority youth are suffering from staggering levels of stress, depression, and physical and mental abuse. These, not surprisingly, often result in higher rates of risky and, therefore, health-compromising behaviors.

Two distressing areas of concern directly related to high-risk behaviors are the alarming rates at which minority adolescents are contracting sexually transmitted diseases and becoming pregnant unintentionally. Approximately one out of eight teenagers in the United States is infected with a sexually transmitted disease every year. This rate is as high as one in four for minority youth in some urban settings (Mosher and Ral, 1991). Chlamydia infection is continually increasing, as are gonorrhea, genital warts, herpes and syphilis. One of the most life-threatening consequences of early unprotected intercourse is infection with the human immunodeficiency virus (HIV). Certain minority groups are disproportionately affected by HIV infection. Through December 1992, the Centers for Disease Control and Prevention had reports of 253,448 AIDS cases. African Americans accounted for almost 30 percent of these cases, nearly 17 percent occurred in Hispanic populations, whereas Asian Americans and Native Americans accounted for fewer than 1 percent combined. Hispanic and African-American youth together account for more than half of all teens and three-quarters of all children infected with HIV. Nationally, almost 84 percent of children with perinatally acquired AIDS are African American or Hispanic, with some states reporting much higher infection and mortality rates. In New York state, for example, AIDS has been the leading cause of death for Hispanic children ages one through four, and the second leading cause of death for African-American children since 1988 (Centers for Disease Control and Prevention, 1993).

Normal feelings of invulnerability and tendencies toward risk taking make adolescents particularly vulnerable to infection with HIV. From 1981 to 1992, the number of reported AIDS cases among 15 to 24 year olds rose from one to 159. By 1989, HIV infection and AIDS had become the sixth leading cause of death for 15 to 24 year olds in the United States. An unsettling aspect of HIV infection is that the latency period between acquiring HIV and exhibiting symptoms of AIDS can be as long as ten years. Currently, one in five of all reported AIDS cases is diagnosed in individuals ages 20 to 29. It can be presumed that many of these individuals acquired HIV during their teenage years (Centers for Disease Control and Prevention, 1993).

Early sexual intercourse places young people, particularly young women, at higher risk for negative health consequences. Youth who begin sexual activity early in life tend to have more partners throughout their lifetime, and are less likely to use effective methods of contraception or protection against sexually transmitted disease. Some of the most severe consequences of early childbearing are the personal effects on these women, their families, and, ultimately, the communities in which they live. Young adolescent mothers suffer more physical strain, with heightened risks of pre- and perinatal complications and mortality. They are more likely to have toxemia, anemia and prolonged labor, and their babies are at higher risk for prematurity and low birth weight. Low birth weight seems to be the strongest risk factor for infant mortality and is most frequently found in African-American newborns, followed by Filipino, Hawaiian, Japanese, and Native-American. The data available for Hispanics suggest a relatively small proportion of low birth weight infants, although this proportion varies depending upon the country of origin. Puerto Ricans have the highest rates of low birth weight babies of all Hispanic populations. African-American, Hispanic,and Native-American women also have higher percentages of preterm births (Dryfoos, 1990; U.S. Department of Health and Human Services, 1992).

The number of single teens becoming pregnant and giving birth has become a growing concern for most of the country. In the past decade, this trend has grown in 42 of the fifty states, and a 14 percent increase has been noted nationally. The percent of low birth weight infants also continues to rise. With these increases come elevated percentages of infants and children who exhibit failure to thrive and latent emotional and/or behavioral consequences (Center for the Study of Social Policy, 1992). Many of the problems encountered by teen mothers mirror those experienced by older mothers who are economically deprived. Postpartum teen mothers tend to have reduced educational achievement, higher divorce rates, more subsequent unintended pregnancies and lower incomes. The combination of these factors often causes the children of very young parents to experience behavioral and emotional difficulties, lower achievement levels, and higher risks of becoming teenage parents themselves. Once this cycle is created, it becomes increasingly difficult to break the chain (Dryfoos, 1990).

In general, having fewer financial resources leaves these families less able to secure the necessary housing, education and health services which encourage and sustain health-promoting behaviors. Reduced incomes usually necessitate longer work hours, resulting in less time for the supervision, education and nurturing of children. Domestic life can become increasingly stressful for these families, resulting in a disturbing entanglement of physical and emotional consequences.

Access to Health Care Services

In addition to health knowledge, the nature of a person's contact with health services is probably the strongest factor affecting health attitudes and subsequent behavior. This contact normally begins in early childhood and is well shaped by adolescence. However, the structural, financial and personal barriers that low-income minority families face when attempting to secure satisfactory health care can easily become transformed into mistrust of health providers, misuse of health delivery systems, and, ultimately, reduced interest in accessing future services. In order to receive health screenings and other wellness care, there must be contact with health services. Intimidation, language, legal status, location of services, hours of operation, finances, and insufficient staff and services, create barriers that are often insurmountable for the populations which they are meant to serve. Not surprisingly, differences in utilization patterns for preventive services are apparent along socioeconomic rather than ethnic or racial lines. The poorest and uninsured in all age and ethnic categories are the least likely to have regular exams and participate in wellness activities sponsored by traditional medical providers (U.S. Department of Health and Human Services, 1992). As a rule, poor youth are less able to identify and therefore utilize sources of health care than their peers from higher socioeconomic households (Klein et al., 1992).

Provider location, hours of operation, disposable income, educational level, cultural beliefs and social values all influence a person's access to health care. Although quantifying levels of access is virtually impossible, several predictors of potential versus realized access have been suggested. Potential access, or the probability that services are available to a given individual, is most directly affected by predisposition, enabling factors and need. The likelihood that an individual will utilize available services results from combined effects of age, gender, ethnicity, education and attitudes. Enabling factors refer to the resources already available to the individual and need refers to the reason for seeking specific services (Aday, Anderson and Fleming, 1980).

Of the 31 million Americans who lack health insurance, nearly 30 percent are minors. One out of every three adolescents below the poverty level has no health insurance. Many insured youth are not covered for preventive care, counseling, substance abuse treatment or other essential services (Newacheck and McManus, 1988; Office of Technology Assessment, 1991). For the average American family, the percent of children who are not covered by any health insurance, including Medicaid, remains steady at approximately 20 percent. For African-American and Hispanic children, this number can be as high as 25 to 35 percent (Center for the Study of Social Policy, 1992).

As evidenced by low socioeconomic status and inadequate insurance, most minority groups lack the ability to access health services, especially primary care. This is troublesome considering the implicit need for preventive care due to high birth rates and young populations. Even with Medicaid and public health clinics, preschool minority children are less likely to be immunized against major childhood diseases. Only 75 percent of preschool children ages one to four are fully immunized; these numbers decrease for minorities in city centers (U.S. Department of Health and Human Services, 1992). For populations living in isolated communities, such as Native Americans, traditional medical delivery systems are ineffective. Unfortunately, the situation is not much better for minorities living in major urban centers with a greater number of health practitioners. Even though title VI of the Public Health Service Act guarantees that health care facilities provide a percentage of uncompensated care to indigent persons, the volume of services delivered through this type of program is insufficient to meet the basic health need of these populations (Aday, Anderson and Fleming, 1980). The net result is overcrowded facilities with overworked staff, limited resources and long waiting times, which act as major deterrents to utilizing available health services. Additional problems in accessing the health care system arise for immigrant groups who lack facility in English or are unfamiliar with and/or have cultural values that conflict with traditional western medical practice. Some of these groups rely on the use of folk medicines for self-treatment as a primary source of health care.

Every minority group (or subgroup) varies in its inclination and need to utilize existing health services. Prenatal care is a prime example of this pattern. It is commonly agreed that prenatal and wellness measures during pregnancy significantly increase the likelihood that a child will thrive during infancy, and that physical and emotional problems will be significantly reduced at a later date. An estimated 20 percent of children ages 3 to 17 suffer from developmental, learning or emotional disorders that are largely preventable in the pre- and perinatal stages. This figure probably understates these problems for minority children whose parents are less likely to report such problems (Zill and Schoenborn, 1990). Despite this, minority women are less likely to receive adequate prenatal care. One-tenth of African-American women do not receive any form of prenatal care and fewer than one-tenth of Native-American women receive prenatal care. In contrast to other minorities, Asian Americans are most likely to receive prenatal care. Overall, less-educated and low-income women are more likely to continue behaviors such as smoking or substance use during pregnancy, which can have grave consequences on infant health. Unfortunately, many minority teens and women fall into this category.

Dental care is another area in which preventive measures are extremely effective. Although dental diseases are rarely life threatening, they can be severely debilitating, resulting in nutritional deficits, systemic infection, disfigurement and financial burdens. According to a recent study, members of larger families, adults who were unemployed or in blue-collar jobs, and those with no private dental insurance have the lowest probability of having regular dental check-ups. Mexican Americans were least likely to utilize dental services, regardless of income or educational levels (Aday, 1992). Most immigrant and many other minority families fall into one or more of these categories. Minority children, particularly Native Americans, tend to have higher rates of dental decay. In general, there are substantially higher unmet needs for dental treatment among African-American, Native-American, and Mexican-American children (Aday, 1992; U.S. Department of Health and Human Services, 1992). This may suggest a need for more school-linked dental programs which reach out to minority children and adults.

Other structural barriers continue to inhibit minorities from entering the health care system. Insufficient or poorly circulated information about available services results in programs which are underutilized and cannot be sustained over time. Issues of confidentiality are of particular concern for adolescents. Fear of deportation and discrimination prevent many new and undocumented immigrants from attempting to seek medical care. Ultimately, children are products of their environment. When adults who care for these children are unable to access sufficient health services, the establishment and maintenance of health-promoting behaviors becomes extremely difficult.

According to the Children's Defense Fund, 700,000 children no longer receive Aid to Families with Dependent Children (AFDC) and Medicaid. Although the need is greater, the percentage of poor children receiving AFDC and Medicaid is much lower than a decade ago (McCuen, 1988). Inadequate preventive care places children at unnecessary risk of poor health. It is estimated that by the year 2000, the United States will have spent in excess of two billion dollars to care for low birth weight infants who require intensive medical intervention to sustain them through the first year of life (Aday, Anderson and Fleming, 1980). Much of this is avoidable with adequate health education and services.

Designing Effective Comprehensive Programs

The heterogeneous nature of ethnic and minority groups makes it difficult to compare health attitudes and behaviors within these groups, and draw comparisons with others. Enormous diversity in attitudes and behaviors exists among and within cultures and subcultures. Educators, administrators and policy-makers need to learn to identify differences in cultural attitudes that influence health behaviors. These might include specific causes of illness, beliefs in the curative powers of people or treatments, the application of modern versus folk medicine principles, and general expectations concerning health. Issues of self-esteem, family structures, gender roles and the effects of personal beliefs and values on health and well-being are central to any quality health education program.

Quality health instruction develops the skills essential for any individual to achieve responsible adulthood. It helps students define themselves, and understand and accept their personal value system. Health instruction fine-tunes problem-solving and decision-making skills, and teaches effective communication and interaction with family, peers and other community members. The tension between the pressure to achieve and the acceptance of peers is addressed, and the potential benefits and consequences associated with specific attitudes, behaviors, and activities are examined (Dryfoos, 1990). Each of these essential aspects of the maturation process are developed and enhanced when comprehensive school health promotion programs are implemented effectively.

In order to reach increasingly disadvantaged and disenfranchised youth and their families, programs must be culturally sensitive, intensive, comprehensive and flexible. They must offer a broad spectrum of services that address multiple needs and view the child in the context of his or her family and the family as part of their community. Skilled and competent staff must coordinate and deliver these programs, which may necessitate larger streams of funding. Staff must be willing to focus on organizational and client objectives to the exclusion of turf issues. In essence, each of the barriers cited previously must be addressed concurrently in order to welcome clients into a user-friendly system. Any truly comprehensive health promotion effort must be supported by effective education programs aimed at reducing the risk for unhealthy lifestyles and behaviors and educational failure.

The fact that a person's culture is dynamic and changes over time with exposure to the popular media and other ethnic and religious groups creates a particular challenge for designing prevention programs for minorities. The cultural diversity present in any community results from the interchange of differing heritages and increases the range of behaviors and beliefs for that community. A thorough understanding of a culturally diverse community can only be achieved through local inquiry and research.

Comprehensive programs designed for minorities must enhance availability, visibility, quality, confidentiality, affordability, flexibility and coordination if they are to encourage regular use by those populations. Services for youth must be age appropriate. The location of service providers and hours of operation should reflect the needs and desires of the target population. The establishment of school-based clinics, transportation to service sites, and extended service hours are potentially effective methods of expanding availability. Great care must be taken to make health services for underserved populations easily recognizable and convenient. Outreach, including education about prevention and how/when to use different services is essential for the success of such programs.

Competent, culturally sensitive professionals must be recruited to practice in programs for underserved populations. Confidentiality should be ensured, both for those persons with questionable immigration status, as well as for adolescents who wish to obtain information and services without parental consent. Public and private programs must provide reimbursement for health promotion activities in addition to required medical interventions. Services, providers and delivery sites must reflect the cultural and social aspects of health that affect the population they serve. Finally, medical, mental health, education and social service providers within the community must effectively coordinate services to provide high quality and continuous care (Klein et al., 1992; Schorr, 1988).

References

Aday, L. A. 1992. A profile of Black and Hispanic subgroups access to dental care: Findings from the National Health Interview Survey. *Journal of Public Health Dentistry* 52 (4): 210-215.

Aday, L. A., R. Anderson and G. Fleming. 1980. *Health care in the United States: Equitable for whom?* New York: Sage Publications.

Center for the Study of Social Policy. 1992. *Kids count data book: State profiles of child well-being.* Washington, DC.

Centers for Disease Control and Prevention. 1993. National AIDS hotline training bulletin February 22 (24).

Centers for Disease Control and Prevention. 1993. National AIDS hotline training bulletin March 19 (36).

Children's Defense Fund. 1985. *A manual on providing effective prenatal care for teens.* Washington, DC.

Dryfoos, J. G. 1990. *Adolescents at risk: Prevalence and prevention.* New York: Oxford University Press.

Grant, C. A. 1988. Race, class, gender, and schooling. *Education Digest* 88: 561-569.

Klein, J. D., G. B. Slap, A. B. Elster and S. K. Schonberg. 1992. Access to health care for adolescents: A position paper of the society for adolescent medicine. *Journal of Adolescent Health* 13 (2): 162-170.

Kolbe, L. J. 1985. Why school health education? An empirical point of view. Presented at the Delbert Oberteuffer Centennial Symposium, Atlanta, GA, April 1985.

Lin-Fu, J. S. 1988. Population characteristics and health care needs of Asian Pacific Americans. *Public Health Reports* 103 (1): 18-27.

McCuen, G. E. 1988. *Poor and minority health care.* Hudson, WI: Gem Publications, Inc.

Mosher, W. D., and S. O. Ral. 1991. Testing for sexually transmitted diseases among women of reproductive age: United States, 1988. *Family Planning Perspectives* 23 (5): 216-221.

National Center for Health Statistics. Examination and health history findings among children and youths, 6-17 years, United States, 1973. Vital and Health Statistics Series 11(129). Washington, DC.

National Education Association. 1989. *The relationship between nutrition and learning.* Washington, DC.

Newacheck, P. W., and M. A. McManus. 1988. Health insurance status of children in the U.S. *Pediatrics* 81:385-394.

Office of Technology Assessment. 1991. *Adolescent health volume I: Summary and policy options.* Washington, DC.

Resnick, M. D., and R. Hibbard. 1988. Chronic physical and social conditions of youth: Study group report. *Journal of Adolescent Health Care* 9:275-325.

Schaffer, D., K. Bacon, P. Fisher, and A. Garland. 1987. *Review of youth suicide prevention programs.* Albany: New York State Task Force on Youth Suicide Prevention.

Schorr, L. B. 1988. *Within our reach.* New York: Anchor Press (Doubleday).

United States Department of Health and Human Services. 1985. Report of the secretary's task force on Black and minority health: Crosscutting issues in minority health, volume 2. Washington, DC.

United States Department of Health and Human Services. 1992. *Health status of minorities and low-income groups.* 3d ed. Washington, DC.

United States Census Bureau. 1990. *Statistical abstract of the United States: 1990.* 110th ed. Washington, DC.

Waller, A. E., S. P. Baker, and A. Szocka. 1989. Childhood injury deaths: National analysis and geographic variations. *American Journal of Public Health* 79 (3): 310-315.

Zill, N., and C. A. Schoenborn. 1990. *Developmental learning and emotional problems: Health of our nation's children, United States, 1988.* Hyattsville, MD: Centers for Disease Control and Prevention.

Chapter 2

The Acculturation Process and Implications for Education and Services

J. Manuel Casas, PhD, and Antonio Casas, MA

The major ethnic groups in the United State, i.e., Hispanic/ Latino, Asian American, African American and American Indian, have received increased attention in social science literature. At the same time there has been an increase of criticism directed at the quality as well as the pragmatic value of this literature. A major criticism has focused on the researchers' failure to accurately define and/or describe the racial/ethnic samples used in their studies (Ponterotto and Casas, 1991). More specifically, this criticism focuses on the prevailing tendency to use what Trimble (1991) has called "ethnic glosses" or overly general labels (e.g., Hispanics) to identify a specific racial/ethnic group while totally ignoring the extensive variables that serve to specifically identify and/or differentiate the individuals who comprise such a group. According to Marín (1992) these variables could include generational history and national background, as well as particular demographic characteristics that may be relevant for a given study, including socioeconomic status, educational attainment and migration history.

A specific psychosocial process that a growing number of researchers believe must be understood and taken into consideration when doing research on racial/ethnic minority populations, especially those who are comprised of a large number of immigrants, is the acculturation process (Ponterotto and Casas, 1991; Trimble, 1991). A major reason for directing attention to this process is the fact that, given all available census information, the major racial/ethnic minority cultural groups will continue to grow at a significant pace as a result of high birth and/or immigration rates (Ponterotto and Casas, 1991). Most culturally sensitive researchers contend that it is very important to take this process into consideration in order to accurately understand and/or interpret the psychosocial makeup (e.g., beliefs, values and attitudes) and behaviors of these individuals, as well as to better understand some of the prevailing problems that exist within these groups. Furthermore, these researchers contend that without this understanding the educational and social service needs of these groups cannot be effectively met.

Underscoring the importance of moving away from an ethnic gloss perspective to one that is more sensitive to the variety of differences that exist within racial/ethnic minority groups, this chapter provides a comprehensive overview of the acculturation process and the models that have been used to explain this process. Attention is then directed to the implications of this process vis-a-vis the psychosocial functioning of racial/ethnic minority individuals. The intention is to provoke thought among educators regarding the vital need to take these processes into consideration in order to design and deliver more culturally sensitive, appropriate and effective services to all persons from diverse racial/ethnic minority backgrounds.

This chapter focuses solely on the acculturation process which is most appropriate for groups who are comprised of a significant number of immigrants. Subsequently, the chapter focuses primarily on Hispanics/Latinos and Asian Americans. Such a focus should in no way be interpreted to mean that other racial/ethnic minority groups do not experience similar or complementary processes as they attempt to adjust in one form or another to the dominant culture in the United States. For example, with respect to African Americans, a more appropriate developmental model that helps to explain their adjustment and adaptation to the mainstream culture is the racial identity developmental model. Unfortunately, we are unable to address this model within the limits of this chapter. Readers interested in getting information relative to this model should refer to Helms (1990). As regards American Indians, we reserve any and all comments relative to the developmental and adaptive processes which they have experienced and are experiencing in the United States. The sad reason for this is that the American Indian population has been all but forgotten by White researchers and, therefore, there is little or no empirical psychological information on this very complex and diverse population.

Acculturation: A General Overview

The concept of acculturation appears as early as 1880; however, the definition which until recently has been most widely accepted was formulated in 1936 by Redfield, Linton and Herskovits (1936). Acculturation is evidenced by those phenomena that result when groups of individuals having different cultures come into continual firsthand contact, with subsequent changes in the original culture patterns of either or both groups.

Unfortunately, this definition largely confined the study of acculturation within the fields of anthropology and sociology. Furthermore, according to Marín (1992), although acculturation did not receive serious research attention within the realm of psychology until the 1970s (Berry, 1974a, 1974b; Brislin, Lonner and Thorndike, 1973; Olmedo, 1979), it is now generally accepted and largely defined as a multidimensional psychosocial phenomenon reflected in psychological changes that occur in individuals as a result of interaction with a new culture.

It is important to distinguish between acculturation and assimilation. Acculturation is generally seen as a change in one culture as a result of contact with another culture, while assimilation is seen as the social, economic and political integration of an ethnic minority cultural group into mainstream society (Keefe and Padilla, 1987). Keefe and Padilla further point out that acculturation must, to some extent, precede assimilation. This stands to reason. After all, to assimilate into a culture one must be able to communicate in the language of the culture as well as understand and be able to emulate the principal values, customs and behaviors inherent in the culture. However, it should not be assumed that movement from acculturation to assimilation is a linear process. There is plenty of historical evidence that shows that acculturation does not ensure assimilation.

For example, Gordon (1964) argues that the experience of many racial/ethnic minorities in the United States who are not of northern European descent has been acculturation without assimilation. One major reason for this is that acculturation as a psychological-sociological phenomena will more than likely occur with or without a planned intent. That is to say, individuals who find themselves submerged in a totally new culture, which cannot be ignored or avoided, will eventually come to tolerate, accept and/or be subsumed into the new culture. It would take a very concerted effort to avoid this result. In contrast, assimilation can be sharply curtailed by discrimination at the individual, institutional or even societal levels. For example, the passage of ethnocentric or racist motivated legislation, such as the Federal Chinese Exclusion Act passed by Congress in 1882, very effectively curtails assimilation.

From a sociological-psychological perspective the construct of acculturation is the product of cultural learning that occurs as a result of contact between the members of two or more groups. Working from this definition, acculturation is then presented as a process of attitudinal and behavioral change undergone, willingly or unwillingly, by individuals who reside in multicultural societies or who come in contact with a new culture due to colonization, invasions or other political changes (Marín, 1992). Furthermore, researchers contend that the psychological and social changes that may occur in the process of acculturation are dependent on the characteristics of the individual (e.g., level of initial identification with the values of the culture of origin), the intensity of and importance given to the contact between the various cultural groups, and the actual numerical balance between individuals representing the original culture and those who represent the new and, more than likely, larger majority culture. Finally, of utmost importance in understanding acculturation from a socio-psychological perspective, is the fact that it is perceived to be an open-ended process.

According to Marín (1992) this attitudinal and behavioral learning that occurs in the acculturation process may be perceived as occurring at three levels:

- The first level, or superficial level, basically involves the learning (and forgetting) of facts that are part of one's cultural history or tradition. At this level, acculturating individuals might begin to forget the names of important historical figures, or other important historically related facts relative to the country of origin, while, in turn, learning prominent historical facts of the culture of the new country in which they find themselves.

- At the second, or intermediate level, the learning that can be expected to take place as a function of acculturation involves the more central behaviors that are perceived to be at the core of a person's social life such as language preferences and use. Furthermore, Marín (1992) contends that other possible indicators of this level of acculturation include ethnicity of friends, neighbors and co-workers, ethnicity of spouse, names given to children, and preference for ethnic media in multicultural environments.

- The third level is referred to as the significant level. At this level, changes take place in the individual's beliefs, values and norms—those essential constructs that prescribe people's world views and interaction patterns. The changes that occur at this level tend to be more permanent and are reflected in the day-to-day activities of the acculturated individual. A number of examples of changes that occur at this level are aptly presented by Marín (1992). One in particular that merits attention here is the change that impacts the traditional value that encourages positive interpersonal relationships and discourages negative, competitive and assertive interactions—what has been called the "simpatía" script (Triandis et al., 1984). According to Marín, the acculturation process can change this social script so that it generally becomes less central to the individual, or, at the very least, becomes a behavioral standard to which attention is given only when the individual is interacting with other, less acculturated Hispanics. Other group-specific values and norms that researchers have shown to be affected by the acculturation process include, but are not limited to, familialism (Sabogal et al., 1987) and collectivism (Marín and Triandis, 1985; Triandis, 1990).

Acculturation Models

While psychologists, sociologists and anthropologists have sought to understand the acculturation process from a general perspective, they have also tried to identify sociopsychological and environmental models from which to better understand the evolution of the process itself. In this section we first direct attention to those models addressed in the literature which have historically received a significant amount of attention. These models include the following: the *dominant majority model,* the *transitional model,* the *alienation model,* the *multidimensional model* and the *bicultural model.* Although it is beyond the scope of this chapter to examine each of these models in detail, a brief overview of each is provided here to give the reader a general understanding of them.

Before providing such an overview, it should be noted that the first three models addressed, the *dominant majority model,* the *transitional model* and the *alienation model,* have been severely criticized due to their overtly or covertly supporting prejudicial attitudes toward individuals who are attempting to acculturate and/or assimilate to the dominant Euro-American society. Each of these models has at some time been adopted by American society as the appropriate belief regarding how groups arriving in the United States *should* fit in. Attention is then directed toward three other models which are presently receiving a great deal of attention by researchers and practitioners alike. These models include the *cultural adaptation model,* the *family biculturalism model* and the *orthogonal cultural identification model.*

The Dominant Majority Model

The dominant majority model, as described by Oetting and Beauvais (1991), has as its goal to have the minority culture adjust to the majority. It tends to be ethnocentric, prejudiced and value laden. Members of the majority culture view themselves as superior while viewing the minority culture as inferior. The acculturation experience of ethnic/cultural minorities was uphill from the "old and bad" to the "new and good." Failure to accept and incorporate the values, beliefs and behaviors of the dominant culture implied weakness and inadequacy.

This model is illustrated in the works of nineteenth-century historical researchers who focused their efforts on writing the history of Texas. Specifically, these historians published research that was seriously flawed in terms of: (1) selectively focusing upon data which perpetuated and reinforced the Euro-American ethnocentric perspective while ignoring other clearly related and relevant data which did not support this perspective; and (2) related to this, focusing upon data which presented a clear bias against Mexicans, especially concerning the relationships between Whites and Mexicans (De León, 1983). Relative to these flaws, De León writes:

> These same historians failed to comment upon an austere Anglo-American moral code that translated the morality of Mexicanos into a defective one, a chauvinistic sentiment that discriminated against un-American nonconformists, and the fact that Texas society placed few social restrictions on a long tradition of violence which ultimately aided and abetted White Texans in keeping ethnic minorities subordinated. (p. *x*)

The Transitional Model

The transitional model (Stonequist, 1964) accepts the minority culture as valuable and attributes any problems encountered by acculturating individuals to the process of moving from one culture to another. There is an implicit assumption within this model that movement toward the majority culture must and will take place. One of the problems that people are assumed to encounter in this model is that of having to make choices relative to their identity. This can be illustrated by the following example provided by Kim (1980):

> Some years ago, my five-year-old son came home from school, shortly after entering kindergarten in a predominantly White neighborhood and asked me: "What am I? Am I Korean or an American?" Trying to be a good mother, I told him he was a Korean American—he was born in the United States of Korean parents, and thus he had a rich heritage from the two cultures. This did not comfort my son, nor did he seem to feel enlightened by the knowledge of his bicultural background. Instead, he protested, "If I am Korean, why can't I speak Korean like you do? And, if I'm an American, how come I don't look like the American kids in my class?" He paused for a moment and then delivered the final blow: "Besides, they call me Chinese!"

Kim further indicates that:

> What's lacking at present—in both school and the home environment—is a conscious articulation of the decisions, choices and comparisons that must be made by the bicultural individual. (p. 101)

The Alienation Model

The alienation model (Graves, 1967) examines the role of alienation that can be experienced by individuals moving toward the majority culture or by individuals who are seeking to establish themselves as bicultural persons. This model compares individuals who are able to function effectively while they are in the transition process to others who are not able to do so. This model emphasizes the perspective that individuals who feel they have the means to achieve the goals valued by the dominant society are able to cope successfully with the transition. If dissonance between the means and/or the goals exists, the person can become alienated from both cultures.

While it provides the individual alternative routes of movement that presumably do not involve stress, this model still contains an implicit assumption that movement towards the dominant culture must and will take place. In the past, this model with its emphasis on alienation has been used to explain gang membership among racial/ethnic minorities (Cohen, 1955). For example, in addressing the issue of alienated youth who may be experiencing difficulties with adjustment and are attracted to the gang subculture, Cohen (1955) contends that the delinquent subculture provides criteria of status which the children can meet in the gangs but may not be able to meet in the broader culture.

The Multidimensional Model

The multidimensional model (Olmedo, Martinez and Martinez, 1978; Olmedo and Padilla, 1978) recognizes the complexity of individuals, and views people in transition along a number of different dimensions including, but not limited to, language preference, social interactions and food preferences. In this model there is less of an assumption that one culture will dominate and that movement towards the dominant culture is essential. Furthermore, in this model, both cultures are valued. Consequently, although there are a number of dimensions involved in the transition, the individual is perceived to exist on a continuum between the two cultures relative to these dimensions.

Related to multiple dimensions is the concept of selective acculturation which has been used to describe the practice of an individual to selectively acculturate more in some dimensions while retaining other traditional cultural values and patterns (Keefe and Padilla, 1987). This can be exemplified by an individual who speaks the English language at work (which may improve socioeconomic status), yet prefers the traditional language at home.

The Bicultural Model

The bicultural model (Ramirez, 1984; Ruiz, Casas and Padilla, 1977) emphasizes that an individual can have simultaneous involvement within two cultures. Ramirez (1984) describes the bicultural/multicultural person as having had extensive socialization and life experiences in two or more cultures and participating actively in these cultures. This model is much broader and more flexible in scope and acknowledges that individuals can identify strongly with more than one culture at any one time. According to this model the individual is on a continuum dependent upon the degree of identification within each culture. This model fails to demonstrate, however, that there may be levels and subtypes of cultural identification within each culture. Bicultural individuals are the result of socialization between two cultures and may be dependent upon both for their ethnic/cultural identification.

Bicultural conceptualization can be understood by discussing the difference between acculturation and ethnic identification. Ethnic identification has been found to be a separate process regardless of the degree of acculturation of the individual (Graves, 1967; Rose, 1964; Rubel, 1966). An individual may have completely acculturated to the majority culture, yet still identify strongly with his or her original culture. For example, Masuda, Matsumoto and Meredith (1970) administered an ethnic identity questionnaire to Japanese Americans in Seattle and Honolulu. They found that although there was a "graded erosion" of Japanese traits over the three generations, there was a considerable retention of ethnic identification even by the third-generation participants.

Of the acculturation models described here, the multidimensional and bicultural models are the only two not viewed as covertly or overtly prejudicial. They are, however, limited in that they do not account for the unique pluralistic cultural patterns which have emerged within ethnic enclaves (Keefe and Padilla, 1987). Furthermore, although the definition of acculturation describes changes in both cultures as the result of continuous first-hand contact, all of these models explicitly or implicitly describe changes which occur to the individual from the minority culture. It is incorrectly assumed that members of the dominant culture do not change or adapt to cultural characteristics of the minority group. Examples of such changes by members of the dominant cultural group can be as subtle as enjoying cultural/ethnic foods and/or celebrating cultural/ethnic events or as overt and complex as marriage between cultures.

Cultural Adaptation Model

A more recent model of acculturation formulated with much detail by Berry (1976a, 1976b, 1988), approaches the acculturation process from an ecological-cultural-behavioral orientation that is essentially based on a perspective of cultural adaptation of the individual to the dominant society. According to Berry, there are four types of adaptations that individuals can choose to make:

Assimilation is defined as the individual relinquishing cultural identity and moving toward the larger society. An example of this is an immigrant who sacrifices his or her original language, cultural customs and even ethnic foods in an attempt to fit into American culture. These individuals are expected to become part of the new group, to "fit in" with the members of the dominant culture.

Integration is defined as the individual maintaining his or her integrity as well as becoming part of the larger society. Integration proposes that individuals learn to react to cultural cues in a culturally appropriate fashion. An example of this is an immigrant who values American culture and has clearly made attempts to fit in, while at the same time maintaining aspects of the original culture which are still valued such as original language, cultural customs and ethnic foods. For example, an individual of Mexican ancestry would act, think and feel as a Mexican when dealing with other Mexicans, but would switch with equal ease to a non-Mexican perspective when interacting with non-Mexicans.

Rejection is defined as the individual withdrawing from the larger society and maintaining his or her cultural identity. Such an individual may live in an ethnic enclave and have little, if any, contact outside of this enclave. Rejection is assumed to take place when individuals choose or are forced to stay separated from the dominant culture—a phenomenon that can take place when segregationist rules or laws are promulgated or when territory is invaded or annexed by another country. For example, Cross (1971) describes Black individuals who choose to completely identify with Black culture and denigrate White culture.

Deculturation is defined as individuals relinquishing cultural identification with their original culture and not attempting to establish relations with the larger society. An example of deculturation are those individuals who seem to have lost touch with their original culture and yet for varied reasons have failed to enter into the new culture.

A weakness inherent in Berry's theory is the implicit assumption that individuals always have the freedom to choose their frame of reference relative to their original culture and/or the larger culture. Adhering to this assumption ignores the negative societal influences that may serve to retard the acculturation process and/or impede the assimilation process. Furthermore, with respect to deculturation, it is hard to imagine an individual making a rational choice to remain marginalized by giving up one culture and choosing not to accept the other culture.

The Family Bicultural Model

Another recent bicultural model of the acculturation process was formulated by Szapocznik, Scopetta, Kurtines and Aranalde (1978). This model addresses acculturation from a psychosocial theoretical perspective and directs attention to the cultural changes and conflicts which may occur within individuals as well as within their respective families. More specifically, these authors propose that acculturation is a complex process of accommodation that may be uni-dimensional or two-dimensional and that when a monocultural context (e.g., an environment in which only the values of the dominant culture are appropriate) prevails, the acculturation process is uni-dimensional and linear as the individual acculturates from the culture of origin to the host culture. They further propose that when a bicultural context (e.g., an environment in which the values of both the original culture and the dominant culture are appropriate) prevails, the acculturation process is two-dimensional and involves an accommodation of the host culture as well as the retention of the culture of origin.

Szapocznik et al. (1978) also propose that the ability of the individual to successfully accommodate to the uni-dimensional or two-dimensional process reflects a normative process of acculturation while a pathological process which deviates from the normative process is reflected in over- or under-acculturation. This deviance is viewed as maladjustment in that it renders the individual inappropriately monocultural in a bicultural context. A normal process of acculturation from within this theoretical perspective is illustrated by Latino immigrants who learn the required behaviors to interact effectively with persons from the larger society while retaining other behaviors that enable them to interact effectively with persons from their original culture.

It should be noted that a major portion of the acculturation research efforts carried out have focused on problem areas, specifically within Latino families, resulting from different levels of acculturation (Szapocznik and Kurtines, 1980; Szapocznik, Kurtines and Fernandez, 1980). Specifically, these researchers have directed attention to problems that arise as a result of the dissonance that can occur when family members acculturate at different speeds.

The Orthogonal Model

The model presently receiving a great deal of attention is the orthogonal model. This model is based upon orthogonal cultural identification theory which contends that identification with different cultures is orthogonal in nature (Oetting and Beauvais, 1991). In essence, this means that identification with any culture is essentially independent of identification with any other culture. In other words, identifying with one culture in no way diminishes the ability of an individual to identify with any other culture. This can be contrasted with all of the preceding models of acculturation which have viewed the individual along a continuum, or continuums between cultures. Orthogonal cultural identification breaks away from this tradition. Orthogonal cultural identification can be understood by visualizing two vectors at right angles to each other with a common beginning point. The origin of the angles represents the lack of identification with any culture, cultural anomie, or cultural alienation. The amount of progression along each of the respective vectors represents the increasing identification of the individual with that culture.

The orthogonal identification model indicates that any pattern combination of cultural identification can exist and that movement or change is possible. Oetting and Beauvais (1991) write:

> A high level of identification with a particular culture should be related to increased probability of engaging in behaviors specific to that culture (or behaviors that

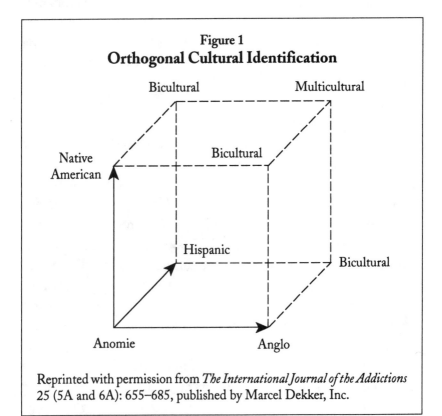

Figure 1
Orthogonal Cultural Identification

Reprinted with permission from *The International Journal of the Addictions* 25 (5A and 6A): 655–685, published by Marcel Dekker, Inc.

the individual believes are part of being in that culture). If for example, an adolescent has a high identification with a minority culture, that should be strongly linked to whether the youth engages in those culture-specific ceremonies or behaviors that are available in the environment. Examples would include religious or initiation ceremonies, family cultural traditions, use of folk medicine, etc. Identification with another culture should have little or no association with these elements of cultural content. (p. 669)

A benefit inherent in this model is the fact that by its very nature it helps reduce the tendency to use "ethnic glosses" or overly general labels to identify persons from specific groups. This is accomplished by stressing the individual's dynamic identification across diverse cultural dimensions instead of being a static part of an ongoing process (Trimble, 1991). The importance of this model lies in identifying important cultural dimensions and variables which are attributes of the individual rather than simply emphasizing his or her ethnic group.

Acculturation and Its Implications to Mental Health and Education

Having provided an overview of the acculturation process and the models that have been used to explain this process, the final section of this chapter directs attention to the implications of the process vis-a-vis the psychosocial functioning of ethnic individuals from diverse ethnic backgrounds. As mentioned at the beginning of this chapter, the purpose of this focus is to provoke thought among educators on the vital need to take this process into consideration if they are to design and deliver more culturally sensitive, appropriate and effective services to all persons. Attention is directed particularly to the implications of the acculturation process with regard to the fields of mental health and education.

Mental Health Implications

From the perspective of mental health, acculturation is customarily seen as an exogenous force shaping psychological distress. More specifically, according to Rogler, Cortes and Malgady (1991) "changes in acculturation entail changes in the person's relationship to the effective environment, which impinges in new ways upon his or her psychological well-being" (p. 588). While there is consensus among researchers that acculturation does have an impact on the psychological functioning of an individual, determining the exact and absolute nature of the impact is still in initial stages of study. For example, it has been hypothesized that acculturation relates statistically and linearly both negatively and positively with psychological distress, also that it relates in a curvilinear fashion to psychological distress, with the result that biculturality produces an optimal mental health situation (Rogler et al., 1991). The arguments underlying these competing predictions that merit serious attention on the part of both researchers and practitioners have been typified in the following ways:

From the perspective of a negative relationship: Immigrants low in acculturation and high in distress have been recently uprooted from traditional supportive interpersonal networks in their society of origin and have not had sufficient time to reconstruct such networks in the host society. Shorn of social bonds, they also experience the strains of pervasive isolation from the cultural parameters of the host society. The strains accumulate in an unfamiliar and unpredictable environment that uncontrollably impinges on everyday life. The absence of instrumental skills, such as knowledge of English, keeps the unfamiliar world from becoming familiar and controllable. Acculturation is low and distress is high. This predicament lowers self-esteem and, eventually, gives rise to the symptomatic behavior (Rogler et al., 1991, p. 588).

From the perspective of a positive relationship: Increases in acculturation alienate the person from traditional supportive primary groups. Increased acculturation also facilitates the internalization of host-society cultural norms, among which may include damaging stereotypes and prejudicial attitudes toward other persons who are a part of the culture of origin. The result of this process is high acculturation and high distress resulting in self-depreciation and ethnic self-hatred in a weakened ego structure. In addition, increases in acculturation expose the person, both socially and ecologically, to the risk of increased alcohol and drug abuse (Rogler et al., 1991, p. 588).

From the perspective of a curvilinear relationship: Good mental health stems from the optimal combination of retaining the supportive and ego-reinforcing traditional cultural elements and learning the host society's instrumental cultural elements. For reasons already mentioned in the two foregoing arguments, psychological distress increases at both acculturative extremes away from the optimal balance point (Rogler et al., 1991, p. 589).

While research findings are mixed relative to supporting any one of the arguments noted above, the lack of methodological consistency across studies makes it impossible to reach any final conclusions. The following findings are from selective studies that have controlled for acculturation:

- There is evidence that gang membership is influenced by marginal integration into both the individual's original culture and/or the contact culture (e.g., the dominant culture of the United States). Gangs permit the development of personal self-identity and identification within the context of multiple marginality (Vigil, 1988).

- There is evidence that "a strong cultural identification should provide a firm and secure base for personal growth and development, provide access to the resources of the culture and limit the potential for serious deviance or violation of cultural norms" (Oetting and Beauvais, 1991).
- Third-generation male adolescents reported higher delinquency rates than either first- or second-generation subjects (Buriel, Calzada and Vazquez, 1982).
- Immigrant Mexican-American adolescents (females and males) reported less alcohol and drug abuse than their White Anglo and second/third generation counterparts (Boles et al., 1993).
- Highly acculturated U.S. born Mexican Americans had higher lifetime prevalence scores of major depression, phobia and dysthymia, as well as higher prevalence of drug and alcohol abuse/dependence than Mexican-born subjects (Burnam et al., 1987; Golding and Karno, 1988; Moscicki et al., 1989).
- Acculturation is associated with decreased abstention among older men and with a higher rate of frequent heavy drinking among younger men. More-acculturated women had five times more probability of being drinkers than women in the low acculturation group. The association between acculturation and alcoholism was stronger for women than for men (Caetano, 1987).
- Mexican-American women in later generations tended to move from light to moderate drinking rates (Gilbert, 1987).
- Best-adjusted Hispanics, as measured by varied psychological scales (e.g., Affect of Balance Scale, Quality of Life Scale), were bicultural, but oriented more toward Hispanic than Anglo culture (Lang et al., 1982).
- Acculturation was significantly associated with higher test scores on the Eating Attitudes Test in the anorexic direction among Hispanic girls (Pumariega, 1986).

- Mexican-American high school student respondents who showed rejection of Mexican-American values reported more difficulties in their relations with their parents (Ramirez, 1969).
- Sex-role traditionalism among Puerto Rican women correlated negatively with assertiveness, and assertiveness correlated negatively with symptoms as measured by the Symptom Checklist–90 (Soto and Shaver, 1982).
- Acculturation levels have also been shown to affect levels of social support (Griffith and Villavicencio, 1985), political and social attitudes (Alva, 1985), health behaviors such as the consumption of cigarettes (Marín, Pérez-Stable and Marín, 1989) and the practice of preventive cancer screening (Marks et al., 1987).
- As levels of acculturation increased, levels of psychological distress also increased among young adults, but not among older individuals (Kaplan and Marks, 1990).

Educational Implications

With respect to education, the number of studies that have given specific attention to acculturation are much fewer. However, given the role that mental health plays in the educational process of children one can extrapolate from the findings in the area of mental health and see how they might relate to the realm of education. The examples presented here are provided to provoke thought among administrators and teachers about the types of programs and practices that might better educate children who find themselves at differing levels in the acculturation process.

- Low-acculturated children may be less likely to assert themselves in the classroom by asking questions and seeking further information and direction that would enable them to successfully accomplish an assignment.
- Recent immigrants, both children and families, who may not

have the social support systems to which they were accustomed in their country of origin may be experiencing significant stress as they navigate the acculturative process (Prieto-Bayard, 1978). Such stress may directly affect their school attendance, and, more specifically, their academic performance.

- Low-acculturated parents may not understand the participatory role that they are expected to play in American schools and because of this may not be actively involved in their children's education. Unfortunately, this lack of involvement has much too often been mistakenly interpreted as a lack of interest in the education of their children.

- Knowing that second-generation Hispanic/Latino youth are more likely to abuse alcohol and other drugs (Boles et al., 1993), educational efforts might be directed towards developing the prevention skills needed by less-acculturated youth to keep their future children from falling prey to alcohol and drugs.

- Knowing that adolescents who retained their Hispanicity but failed to learn adaptive "Americanized" behaviors showed low levels of adjustment (Szapocznik, Kurtines and Fernandez, 1980) might serve as an impetus to provide classes that help newcomers navigate the unfamiliar social and educational systems in which they find themselves. In other words, it would be helpful to provide positive support and direction to individuals who are navigating through the acculturation process.

- Knowing that low-acculturated children may view the learning process from a collectivistic perspective in which they cooperate as a group rather than compete with others should induce teachers to understand and address different styles of learning.

Conclusion

While the concept of acculturation appears relatively early in the social sciences, attention directed to the concept by psychologists is a more recent phenomenon. A major reason for this increased attention is the need to get beyond "ethnic glosses" in order to more accurately understand, and, in turn, effectively service the diversity of individuals who comprise the rapidly growing racial/ethnic minority populations. To this end, the last two decades have seen the development of varied models to help explain the acculturation process. Reflecting the evolutionary process of model building, the earliest models were quite simplistic while the more recent models are much more complex and provide a richer basis from which to understand and appreciate the intricate process of acculturation and all its ramifications. Though not covered in this chapter, it should be noted that concomitant with the development of the models was the development of numerous complementary instruments which enabled researchers to measure and identify the acculturation level of individuals from similar and/or diverse racial/ethnic minority groups. The development of such instruments has been a great boon to the inclusion of acculturation as an important independent variable in a myriad of studies including those that are noted above.

Acculturation must be seen as a valid construct to be taken into serious consideration in the development of research efforts concentrated on ethnically diverse populations. Accepting and understanding this fact will help educators, mental health providers and social service agents to sharpen their focus. This move away from the tendency to use ethnic glosses will enhance efforts to provide more effective and culturally relevant services and programs.

References

Alva, S. A. 1985. Political acculturation and Mexican American adolescents. *Hispanic Journal* of Behavioral Sciences 7:345-364.

Berry, J. W. 1988. *Acculturation and psychological adaptation: A conceptual overview.* In *Ethnic psychology: Research and practice with immigrants, native peoples, ethnic groups and sojourners,* ed. J. W. Berry and R. C. Annis, 41-52. Berwyn, PA: Swets North America, Inc.

Berry, J. W. 1976a. Individual adaptation to change in relation to cultural complexity and psychological differentiation. Paper presented to American Anthropological Association.

Berry, J. W. 1976b. *Human ecology and cognitive style: Comparative studies in cultural and psychological adaptation.* New York: Sage/Halsted.

Berry, J. W. and R. C. Annis. 1974a. Acculturative stress: The role of ecology, culture and differentiation. *Journal of Cross-Cultural Psychology* 5:382-405

Berry, J. W. and R. C. Annis. 1974b. Ecology, culture and psychological differentiation. *International Journal of Psychology* 9:173-193.

Boles, S., J. M. Casas, M. Furlong, L. Gonzalez and G. Morrison. 1993. *Alcohol and other drug use among Mexican American, Mexican and Anglo adolescents: New directions for assessment and research.* (Manuscript submitted for publication.)

Brislin, R. W., W. J. Lonner and R. M. Thorndike. 1973. *Cross-cultural research methods.* New York: John Wiley and Sons.

Buriel, R., S. Calzada and R. Vasquez. 1982. The relationship of traditional Mexican-American culture to adjustment and delinquency among three generations of Mexican-American male adolescents. *Hispanic Journal of Behavioral Sciences,* 4 (1): 41-55.

Burnam, M. A., R. L. Hough, M. Karno, J. I. Escobar and C. A. Telles. 1987. Acculturation and lifetime prevalence of psychiatric disorders among Mexican Americans in Los Angeles. *Journal of Health and Social Behavior* 28:89-102.

Caetano, R. 1987. Acculturation and drinking patterns among U.S. Hispanics. *British Journal of Addiction* 82:789-799.

Casas, J. M. 1984. *Policy, training and research in counseling psychology: The racial/ethnic minority perspective.* In *Handbook of counseling psychology,* ed. S. D. Brown and R. Lent, 785-831. New York: John Wiley and Sons.

Cohen, A. K. 1955. *Delinquent boys: The culture of the gang.* Glencoe, IL: Free Press.

The Multicultural Challenge in Health Education

Cromwell, V. L., and R. W. Cromwell. 1978. Perceived dominance in decision making and conflict resolution among Anglo, Black and Chicano couples. *Journal of Marriage and the Family* 40:749-759.

Cross, W. E., Jr. 1971. The Negro to Black experience: Toward a psychology of Black liberation. *Black World* 20 (9): 13-27.

De León, A. 1983. *They called them greasers: Anglo attitudes toward Mexicans in Texas, 1821–1900.* Austin, TX: University of Texas Press.

Gilbert, M. J. 1987. Alcohol consumption patterns in immigrant and later generation Mexican-American women. Special issue: Mexican immigrant women. *Hispanic Journal of Behavioral Sciences* 9 (3): 299-313.

Golding, J. M., and M. Karno. 1988. Gender differences in depressive symptoms among Mexican Americans and non-Hispanic Whites. *Hispanic Journal of Behavioral Sciences* 10: 1-19.

Gordon, M. M. 1964. *Assimilation in American life: The role of race, religion and national origins.* New York: Oxford Press University.

Graves, D. T. 1967. Acculturation, access and alcohol in a tri-ethnic community. *American Anthropologist* 69: 306-321.

Griffith, J., and S. Villavicenio. 1985. Relationships of acculturation, sociodemographic characteristics and social support in Mexican-American adults. *Hispanic Journal of Behavioral Sciences* 7: 75-92.

Helms, J. E. 1990. *Black and white racial identity: Theory research and practice.* New York: Greenwood Press.

Kaplan, M. S., and G. Marks. 1990. Adverse effects of acculturation: Psychological distress among Mexican-American young adults. *Social Science and Medicine* 31:1313-1319.

Keefe, S. E., and A. M. Padilla. 1987. *Chicano Ethnicity.* Albuquerque, NM: University of New Mexico Press.

Kim, B. L. C. 1980. *Korean-American child at school and at home.* Technical Report to the Administration for Children, Youth and Families. Washington, DC.

Lang, J. G., R. F. Muñoz, G. Bernal and J. L. Sorenson. 1982. Quality of life and psychological well-being in a bicultural Latino community. *Hispanic Journal of Behavioral Sciences* 4 (4): 433-450.

Marín, G. 1992. Issues in the measurement of acculturation among Hispanics. In *Psychological testing of Hispanics* ed. K. F. Geisinger, 235-251. Washington, DC: American Psychological Association.

Marín, G., E. J. Pérez-Stable and B. V. Marín. 1989. Cigarette smoking among San Francisco Hispanics: The role of acculturation and gender. *American Journal of Public Health* 79:196-198.

Marín, G., and H. C. Triandis. 1985. Allocentrism as an important character-istic of the behavior of Latin Americans and Hispanics. In *Cross-cultural and national studies in social psychology,* ed. R. Diaz-Guerrero, 85-104. Amsterdam: Elsevier Science Publishers.

Marks, G., J. Solis, J. L. Richardson, L. M. Collins, L. Birba and J. C. Hisserich. 1987. Health behavior of elderly Hispanic women: Does cultural assimilation make a difference? *American Journal of Public Health* 77:1315-1319.

Masuda, M., G. H. Matsumoto and G. M. Meredith. 1970. Ethnic identity in three generations of Japanese-Americans. *The Journal of Social Psychology* 81:199-207.

Moscicki, E. K., B. Z. Locke, D. S. Rae and J. H. Boyd. 1989. Depressive symptoms among Mexican Americans: The Hispanic Health and Nutri-tion Examination Survey. *American Journal of Epidemiology* 130:348-360.

Oetting, E. R., and F. Beauvais. 1991. Orthogonal cultural identification theory: The cultural identification of minority adolescents. *The International Journal of the Addictions* 25 (5A and 6A): 655-685.

Olmedo, E. L., J. L. Martinez and S. R. Martinez. 1978. Measure of accultura-tion for Chicano adolescents. *Psychological Reports* 42: 159-170.

Olmedo, E. L., and A. M. Padilla. 1978. Empirical and construct validation of a measure of acculturation for Mexican Americans. *Journal of Social Psychology* 105:179-187.

Olmedo, E. L. 1979. Acculturation: A psychometric perspective. *American Psychologist* 34:1061-1070.

Ponterotto, J. G., and J. M. Casas. 1991. *Handbook of racial/ethnic minority counseling research.* Springfield, IL: Charles C. Thomas Publisher.

Prieto-Bayard, M. 1978. *Ethnic identity and stress: The significance of sociocultural context.* In *Family and Mental Health in the Mexican American Community. Monograph no. 7,* ed. J. M. Casas and S. E. Keefe. Spanish Speaking Mental Health Research Center. University of California, Los Angeles.

Pumariega, A. J. 1986. Acculturation and eating attitudes in adolescent girls: A comparative and correlational study. *Journal of the American Academy of Child Psychiatry* 25 (2): 276-279.

Ramirez, M. 1969. Identification with Mexican-American values and psycho-logical adjustment in Mexican-American adolescents. *International Journal of Social Psychiatry* 15:151-156.

Ramirez, M., III. 1984. *Assessing and understanding biculturalism-multiculturalism in Mexican-American adults.* In *Chicano Psychology,* ed. J. L. Martinez and R. H. Mendoza. New York: Academic Press.

Redfield, R., R. Linton and M. J. Herskovits. 1936. Memorandum for the study of acculturation. *American Anthropologist* 38:149-152.

Rogler, L. H., D. E. Cortes and R. Malgady. 1991. Acculturation and mental health status among Hispanics. *American Psychologist* 46:585-597.

Rose, P. I. 1964. *They and we: Racial and ethnic relations in the United States.* New York: Random House.

Rubel, A. J. 1966. *Across the tracks: Mexican Americans in a Texas City.* Austin: Hogg Foundation of Mental Health, University of Texas Press.

Ruiz, R. A., J. M. Casas and A. M. Padilla. 1977. *Culturally relevant behavioristic counseling.* Occasional paper no. 5. Los Angeles: Spanish Speaking Mental Health Research Center, University of California, Los Angeles.

Sabogal, R., G. Marín, R. Otero-Sabogal, B. V. Marín and E. J. Pérez-Stable. 1987. Hispanic familialism and acculturation: What changes and what doesn't? *Hispanic Journal of Behavioral Sciences* 9:397-412.

Soto, E. and P. Shaver. 1982. Sex-role traditionalism, assertiveness and symptoms of Puerto Rican women living in the United States. *Hispanic Journal of Behavioral Sciences* 4 (1): 1-19.

Stonequist, E. V. 1964. *The marginal man: A study in personality and culture conflict.* In *Contributions to urban sociology,* ed. E. Burgess and D. J. Bogue. Chicago: University of Chicago Press.

Sue, S. and J. K. Morishima. 1988. *The mental health of Asian Americans.* San Francisco, CA: Jossey-Bass Publishers.

Szapocznik, J. and W. Kurtines. 1980. Acculturation, biculturalism and adjustment among Cuban Americans.In *Acculturation: Theory, models and some new findings,* ed. A. M. Padilla, 139-160. Boulder, CO: Westview Press.

Szapocznik, J., W. Kurtines and T. Fernandez. 1980. Biculturalism involvement in Hispanic-American youths. *International Journal of Intercultural Relations* 4:353-375.

Szapocznik, J., M. A. Scopetta, W. Kurtines and M. A. Aranalde. 1978. Theory and measurement of acculturation. *Interamerican Journal of Psychology* 12:113-130.

Triandis, H. C. 1990. Toward cross-cultural studies of individualism and collectivism in Latin America. *Interamerican Journal of Psychology/Revista Interamerica de Psicología* 24:199-210.

Triandis, H. C., G. Marín, J. Lisansky and H. Betancourt. 1984. Simpatía as a cultural script of Hispanics. *Journal of Personality and Social Psychology* 47:1363-1375.

Trimble, J. 1991. Ethnic specification, validation prospects and the future of drug use research. *International Journal of the Addictions* 25 (2A): 149-170.

Vigil, J. D. 1988. *Barrio gangs: Street life and identity in Southern California.* Austin, TX: University of Texas Press.

Chapter 3

Ethnicity and the Health Belief Systems

Leonard Jack, Jr., PhD,
Ira E. Harrison, PhD, MPH, and
Collins O. Airhihenbuwa, PhD, MPH

According to the U.S. census, between 1970 and 1980, the total population of diverse racial and ethnic groups increased by 36 percent (i.e., Hispanic Americans, African Americans, Asian Americans, Native American Indians, and Alaskan Natives). In the United States, culturally diverse populations comprise more than 50 percent of the population in 25 cities, numerous counties and the state of California. Recognizing the irreversible fact that in the twenty-first century racial and ethnic groups in the United States will surpass Anglo/Northern Europeans for the first time, school systems will need to address the role ethnicity and culture plays in the health decision-making process.

Several studies, including the Report of the Secretary of Health and Human Services' Task Force on Black and Minority Health (1985), report that low-income culturally diverse populations have limited availability to health services and access to quality care.

With regard to prevention, ethnic minority populations are less likely to be exposed to consistent, quality health promotion programs in their communities and schools (Dorfman, 1990).

School systems across the United States are composed of many ethnic, religious, cultural and socioeconomic groups. Such diversity has made it possible to learn about similarities and differences among groups, recognizing and accepting that a desire for understanding is needed. Similarities and differences are manifested in life experiences, family backgrounds, individual beliefs, attitudes, practices, socioeconomic status, environmental surrounding, etc. These similarities and differences (e.g., life experiences, family influences, beliefs, attitudes and practices) influence health outcomes regardless of ethnicity.

Health itself is a complex issue. In an effort to understand this complex issue, many postulates have been proposed to explain why individuals make certain health decisions in response to the social and environmental context in which people interact and conduct everyday living. Behavioral scientists, including health educators and school officials, are interested in the role ethnicity plays in the decision-making processes of youth in America.

While ethnicity alone may not determine health beliefs, attitudes and practices shared among members of the same ethnic group, it is important to examine health beliefs as they relate to common origins, customs and styles of living within a given ethnic group. This chapter is designed to increase understanding of cultural aspects of health and illness in order to assist with developing more effective and culturally appropriate health education programs for various ethnic groups that have unique and independent cultural beliefs, attitudes and practices.

Cultural Beliefs and Practices

Ethnicity refers to social aggregates which are distinguished primarily by common cultural characteristics (Jack and Airhihenbuwa, 1992). Cultural identity is primarily based on any combination of shared historical, linguistic and psychological lineage (Diop, 1991). These sets of collective factors in a culture influence the group's design for living, the shared set of socially transmitted perceptions about the nature of the physical, social and spiritual world, particularly as they relate to achieving life's goals (Paul, 1955). The differences as well as the similarities of cultural values and perceptions must be carefully examined when developing health education programs in order to appropriately address preventive health behaviors within the context of the mosaic of cultures in the United States (Airhihenbuwa et al., 1992).

Health education and behavior change programs should be developed within the context of diversity in the population (a salad bowl rather than a melting pot). Therefore, programs should be adapted in such a way as to be consistent with the cultural framework of the target community rather than that of the presumed majority American culture within which most programs are developed (Airhihenbuwa and Pineiro, 1988).

Working with various ethnic groups does not require that each respective ethnic group conform to a common pattern of norms or customs (Jack et al., 1993). Instead, mutual respect and understanding is needed from members of different groups with varying culture-bound values desiring to work together (Bailey, 1987). Culture-bound values are used to judge normality and abnormality among various ethnic groups (Sue and Sue, 1977). Culture may be viewed as a learned and transmitted blueprint for living that guides a particular group's thoughts and actions (Jones, 1972). Culture affects many aspects of an individual's daily life. It defines the parameters within which most functions and actions occur. These include thinking and acting, male and female roles, hierarchies of respect, how one acts in groups, other aspects of social relationships, the general outlook on the world, and orientation to time and to the future (Roberson, 1989). Culture also influences the appropriate approaches for prevention and treatment of illness (Jack et al., 1993), hence social and environmental factors must be considered when planning school-based health education programs (Airhihenbuwa, 1992).

Educators must have an understanding of how ethnic groups see themselves despite how they may be grouped or classed by others. In this instance, educators must hear from the ethnic groups they attempt to reach in order to discover ways to ensure acceptance, participation and lifestyle changes by proposed school-based health education programs. In most cases, national surveys examining knowledge, attitudes, beliefs and behaviors are used to design school-based health education programs for various ethnic groups (Roberson, 1989). Research involving youth reveals ethnicity as a salient factor in the way adolescents and younger children conceptualize health and illness.

Cultural Health Beliefs, Attitudes and Practices Among Selected Ethnic Groups

It is critically important to remember that no cultural group is homogeneous, and that every ethnic group contains great diversity (Randall-David, 1989). Cultural universals, structures or functions that are found in every culture (e.g., family units, marriage, parental roles, education, health care, forms of work or endeavors to meet basic physiological needs, and forms of self-expression that meet psychological and spiritual needs) (Radcliffee-Brown, 1935). According to Randall-David (1989), these cultural universals have an impact on issues relating to family roles and relationships, health beliefs about chronic illness and disability, religious beliefs and their interrelationship with health beliefs, food choices, sexual attitudes and practices, drug usage patterns, and styles of communication that affect education.

Persons working with diverse populations ought to remember the 3Rs of good human relations: recognition, respect and relating. They must recognize that today's school populations, especially in metropolitan areas, are more diverse than those of the past. The recognition of this fact should lead to a respect and understanding of differences. Respect means that school officials should accept the challenge to relate to these diverse groups of youth. Relating entails a sensitivity to at least four aspects of ethnic diversity: communication, folk health, spirituality and discrimination.

Folk health, the beliefs and behaviors various groups employ to maintain wellness, order and togetherness, is important for sympathetic communication and intervention with diverse groups. Spirituality, a feeling of connectiveness to and with a higher power, ancestors, special leadership, and special locations (Earth, sky, water) is important for empathetic and insightful relations. Discrimination, or adverse actions experienced by diverse populations, including exclusion from choice residential areas, restriction on reservations and/or plantations, derogatory name calling, labeling, surveillance and policing, must be recognized as areas of pain and psychological distress that may become barriers to well-planned health and educational services.

Examining cultural beliefs, attitudes and practices among specific ethnic groups can assist health education planners in understanding the diversity that exists in a multicultural classroom. To illustrate this statement, examples of characteristics for African Americans, Asian Americans, Mexican Americans and Native

Americans will be briefly discussed. Application of these characteristics should be used with caution given the diversity existing within each ethnic group. However, they can be used as a means of understanding and accepting differences and similarities among ethnic groups.

African Americans

Sensitive communication is crucial to interacting with African Americans. African-American English versus Standard English does not have to be a problem in communication. School officials can work toward understanding the differences, and register a willingness to work with the speaker, rather than deprecate the speech. Focus the student on what is necessary in understanding the health message rather than attempting to alter speech patterns. Speech pattern differences do not indicate lack of intelligence, an unwillingness to learn, or speech disorders (Hall and Harrison, 1993). Derogatory terms such as "you people" can become barriers to meaningful communication.

Folk health among African Americans is centuries old, surviving in folklore, medicine and religion (Harrison, 1975/76). Folk healers (e.g., spiritualists, herbalists) exist, and may be more emotionally, financially and physically accessible than doctors, nurses and pharmacists for attention, cure, treatment and reassurance. School officials should neither condone nor condemn folk healers—a student's relative may be such a healer. Terms like root work, voodoo, hoodoo, fix, mojo, conjuring and hex ought not to cause problems for school officials as they are alternative methods to deal with health, disappointment, death and/or disease.

Spirituality among African Americans centers around the idea of soul. Soul is the essence of life that connects one African American with another. It is positive, persuasive and physical; an emotional, physical bond is claimed by most African Americans as an affirmation of their distinctness (Gwaltney, 1980; Hannerz, 1969).

Spirituality also means religion: the recognition and worship of power beyond oneself. Thus, religious leaders may be both a source and a resource in relating to youth with health messages. They may bring the necessary people together, or they may be able to help gain access to other community leaders (Harrison, 1992). The potential of the African-American preacher to contribute positively to health and educational efforts is not to be minimized.

Discrimination is a fact of life for all African Americans. Words like inner-city, ghetto and bussing are buzzwords illustrating differential treatment accorded African Americans. Historic discrimination in health care has not only meant little or no medical care (Harrison and Harrison 1971; Smith, 1993); but also implied that one is not sick until one sees blood or feels pain. Preventive health and the use of health screening is almost unknown (Bailey, 1991). A person could have hypertension or diabetes yet experience little or no pain. Pain may be blotted out because a person just does not want to be sick and risk the indignities of racial discrimination while engaging in health seeking behavior (Harrison, 1968; Bailey, 1991). Thus, discrimination has led to denial. Denial, whether of HIV/AIDS (Jack and Airhihenbuwa, 1992, Airhihenbuwa, Jack and Wang, 1991; Jack, 1988a; Jack, 1988b) alcoholism, drug abuse (Airhihenbuwa and Jack, 1988; Airhihenbuwa and Pineiro, 1988), hypertension, etc., can be a huge barrier to using preventive or remedial health measures. Finally, the infamous Tuskegee Study (Jones, 1981), in which African Americans were used as guinea pigs, does little to engender faith or hope in the mainstream medical system and, as a result, many African Americans are in advanced stages of disease by the time they are seen by a physician.

Asian Americans

Asian Americans represent a diverse population that includes Chinese, Japanese, Koreans, Filipinos, Southeast Asians and Pacific Islanders. Among each of these groups there is considerable diversity. Variations of languages exist within all groups and within each language are multiple variations of dialect. Each language and dialect is unique and can serve as a facilitator or barrier to participation, comprehension and compliance in any health education program or medical regimen. For example, among Filipinos, the largest population of Asian Americans (Frank-Stromborg and Olsen, 1993), a mixture of Tagalog with Malayo-Indonesian, Chinese, Spanish and English words is used (Lin-Fu, 1988). For this reason, it becomes crucial to involve adult Asian Americans in school systems where Asian-American students attend.

Asian Americans in general have relied on herbs to maintain health or for treatment of illnesses. Among those commonly used are ginseng, honeysuckle flower, Chinese yam, garlic and many others. Traditional medicine has included the use of several techniques that are effective and consistent with Asian-American customs and beliefs, and should not be overlooked or minimized. These techniques include acupuncture, massage, cupping (injecting heat into a cup placed over a body part needing healing), skin scraping (rubbing a coin or blunt smooth object dipped in water or oil on the skin in a back and forth motion), and moxibustion (placing a burning moxa plant directly onto the skin for healing (Frank-Stromborg and Olsen, 1993). Many of these methods are believed to be effective against such diseases as arthritis, stomachaches, abscesses, hypertension, colic and abdominal pain.

The deliverer of health messages and health care is of even greater importance in this population. For each subgroup, special attention should be given to involving appropriate family members to reinforce health messages within the family. While the women may be the caretakers, in some subgroups men reinforce the desired behavior. When it is not possible to include both men and women, it is crucial to be able to target the individual who reinforces behavior in the family. Such an individual may be the only effective educator to address issues of mental and emotional illness among many Asian Americans. Some Asian Americans will go to great lengths to avoid public embarrassment and shame over what may appear as difficulty in role performance, marital problems, or more serious mental disorders (Kunz, et al., 1980; Kemp, 1985; Flaskerud and Soldevilla, 1986).

Some Asian Americans feel that diet is closely associated with health and that illness can be a result of bad conduct within the family. They further believe that medical intervention may interfere with spirituality and that illness and disease occur because of fate (Burney, et al., 1989; Drachman, 1992). While religious practices vary, place of worship appears to be very important to members of this group. Traditional healers may be enlisted to treat emotional disorders and any physical conditions thought to be caused by spirits. Many Asian-American subgroups believe in the law of opposites, "Yin-Yang," or "hot-cold," and also employ dermabrasive procedures to treat health problems. Specifically, the Chinese concept of Yin and Yang means opposite forces that must remain in balance in order to ensure healthy body, mind and spirit. Yang is represented by light, strength, and heat, while Yin is represented by darkness, softness and cold (Frank-Stromborg and Olsen, 1993). Foods and drugs are divided into categories (cold or hot) and are recognized by their properties and believed to have certain effects on health. These beliefs regarding Yin and Yang must be understood and respected given the impact both have on all dimensions of an individual's growth.

Some Asian Americans have become acculturated to Western traditions and practices. However, many have suffered tremendous economic hardships, racial abuse and ethnic acculturation (Drachman, 1992). In addition, Asian Americans have suffered tremendous psychological and physical stress from wars and from being held in concentration camps against their will. Families were separated and females abused physically and emotionally. Many Asians in the United States are refugees from war situations generating fear, displacement and mistrust in a system that will not benefit them. This has major implications regarding the level of acceptance a non-Asian-American person will have in a community. As with other ethnic groups, it is necessary to actively recruit Asian Americans into school systems where members of this population are in attendance.

Mexican Americans

Since Mexican Americans are the nation's second largest minority, discussions of cultural patterns of Mexican Americans will be discussed as a model for other Latinos/Hispanics. However, the authors realize that there is great diversity among Hispanics and Mexican Americans.

Because people more often tend to speak in the language spoken by their parents and siblings, Mexican Americans tend to speak Spanish more frequently than English. Therefore, school officials lacking knowledge of Spanish and/or Latin American culture may themselves be a barrier to health and education efforts among Mexican Americans. Where Spanish fluency is lacking, translators, native Spanish speakers who can translate Spanish into English and English into Spanish quickly and correctly, may be helpful. However, a bilingual, bicultural school official would greatly reduce this barrier.

To understand communication patterns among Mexican Americans, it is important to consider that status and roles are well defined and based on age and gender. Although traditionally the male has more authority than the female in the family, it is the woman who is the nurturer and the information seeker, taking care of family health, education and welfare activities.

There is strong identification with the extended family and often this includes *comadres* and *compadres,* and *madrinas* and *padrinos,* i.e., family friends who become part of the family by baptizing children or witnessing the marital vows at the wedding.

Other values to consider when communicating with Mexican-American families are *respeto,* a deference or deep respect and courtesy shown to others, establishing *confianza,* or trust, and *simpatía,* avoiding conflict and attempting to smooth things over and make communication as positive as possible (Martinez, 1978; Marín, 1991). Knowing the focus of health and welfare activities and understanding the ideal pattern of communication may provide school officials with insights on the difficulties connected with trying to obtain an immediate opinion in a health emergency.

Mexican Americans, like most people, have their own categories of diseases, healers and remedies. School officials should be aware that among very traditional and most often low-income families, *brujeria* (witchcraft) may be a source of ill health. *Mal puesto* (hex), *mal de ojo* (evil eye), *empacho* (indigestion, surfeit), and *susto* (fright) are real disorders to many traditional Mexican Americans. The use of herbs and teas for healing are common remedies to some for these disorders.

Many Mexican Americans are Catholic. This means that mass, baptism, communion, confirmation and confession are important occasions in the lives of many Mexican-American families. The struggle between good and evil may mean that disequilibrium in human relations or the wrath of deities leads to disorder and disease. Praying, celebrating the sacraments and promising *mandas* can be preventive health methods.

Some Mexican Americans are Protestant. Those who are Pentecostal, like many African Americans (Harrison 1971), believe that possession by the Holy Spirit can lead to better health as one is sanctified and saved. School officials working with Mexican-American families might find religious leaders, priests, preachers or prophets, valuable as allies in health care matters.

Finally, discrimination is no stranger to Mexican Americans. Most families are segregated, insulted and isolated into barrios due to exclusionary real estate practices, limited financial means, and/or their desire to live with others who speak Spanish and share Hispanic culture (Clark, 1959; Martinez, 1978). Vèlez-Ibàñez and Greenberg (1992) remind us that U.S. Mexican households have "funds of knowledge" which health and education officials can use to join forces with Mexican Americans to better understand and serve them.

Native Americans

The Native American population is the smallest of the ethnic minority groups in the United States. Currently Native Americans reside in thirty states on reservations and 17 states off reservations (Frank-Stromborg and Olsen, 1993). There are many tribes, each having a distinct language, history and cultural heritage. Some tribes, Apache, Yaqui, Hopi and Navajo tribes for example, speak varying languages which have been influenced by accommodating to Western society. There are many populations that have been forced to exist in bicultural environments. Since European settlement of North America, the traditional mores and cultural patterns of Native Americans have been severely disrupted. Hence, considerable variation exists regarding health beliefs, practices, etc. What appears to be universal among them is that their beliefs about health are closely linked to spiritual beliefs.

Spirituality is very important to this population. As a result, health cannot be separated from spirituality (Randall-David, 1989).

Illness may be viewed as being "unbalanced," caused by natural and/or supernatural forces. Approaches to healing may involve traditional practices that include rituals by a recognized and accepted medicine man.

In this instance, there is a respect for traditional approaches to health despite the availability of other forms of health care. According to Locust (1985, 1987a, 1987b), traditional healing is grounded in several beliefs among Native Americans:

- Native Americans believe in a supreme creator.
- A person is a threefold being made up of body, mind and spirit.
- The spirit existed before it came into a physical body and will exist after the body dies.
- Plants and animals, like humans, are part of the spirit world.
- Wellness is harmony in body, mind and spirit.
- Unwillingness is caused by disharmony between the body, mind and spirit.
- Natural unwillingness is caused by the violation of a sacred or tribal taboo.
- Unnatural unwillingness is caused by witchcraft.
- Each of us is responsible for our own wellness.

Planners of health education programs should recognize that many Native Americans believe they are responsible for their own health or illness. Therefore, this philosophy must be incorporated into program activities and should involve respected Native Americans from this population in the translation of sensitive health messages. The participation of Native Americans in the classroom is of particular importance considering that many Native Americans have not been able to interface with mainstream society.

Unemployment and poverty are extremely high among this ethnic group and have contributed to their isolation in the United States. Historically, Native Americans have experienced poor health resulting from limited prevention and medical resources. As a result of societal alienation and other factors (e.g., poverty, unemployment, fragmented family structures), alcoholism is extremely high. Communication about alcoholism and other illnesses among Native Americans should involve storytelling, an oral tradition. Storytelling is usually done by an older member, particularly where increased age warrants greater respect among members.

Implications for Health Education in the Multicultural Classroom

With such diversity among individual ethnic groups, educators, health professionals and school officials should address the following key questions before developing health education programs:

- What are the health beliefs, attitudes and practices shared among each ethnic group being targeted for health education programs within the school system?
- What impact does ethnicity have on cultural health beliefs, attitudes and practices among ethnic groups to be targeted?
- What key social, economic, political and environmental factors should be taken into consideration when developing health education programs for each ethnic group?
- In what ways are health belief systems reinforced by members of the family, neighborhood and school?
- How are decisions regarding health made by respective ethnic groups?
- Beyond hired school personnel, who should be involved in the planning of health education programs for ethnic groups?
- What are the most appropriate settings in which to conduct health education programs?
- Are school staff representative of the population to be served?

- How will educators, health professionals and school officials be trained to become sensitive to the health beliefs, attitudes and practices among ethnic groups being targeted?

The PEN-3 Model

To address each of these complex questions, educators, health professionals and school officials should employ the use of a comprehensive model that can be used as a guide to ensure that the needs of each ethnic group are met. In 1990, Airhihenbuwa proposed the PEN-3 model, a culturally appropriate method for developing, implementing and evaluating health education for diverse populations (see Figure 1). In the PEN-3 model, it is

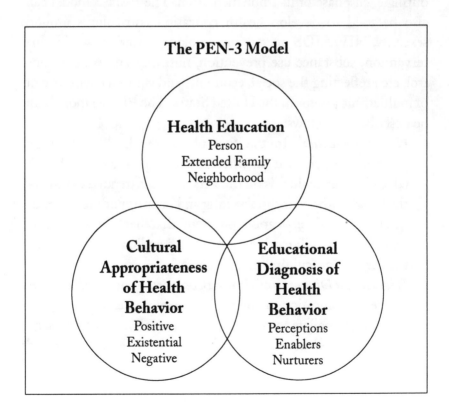

recommended that culturally-based health beliefs respond best to small groups (i.e., school systems, communities, etc.) rather than the media. Media efforts have proven effective only in changing behaviors and beliefs that are newly acquired and/or superficially grounded in culture. The model consists of three dimensions of health beliefs and behaviors that are interrelated and interdependent: **Health Education, Educational Diagnosis of Health Behavior** and **Cultural Appropriateness of Health Behavior.** These dimensions of the model are categorized according to the acronym PEN for each of the three dimensions.

The PEN-3 model has been used in African-American settings and can be used within multiethnic settings as well. This model encourages involvement from the respective ethnic groups during each phase of its implementation. The PEN-3 model can also be used to develop health education curriculums around sexuality, HIV/AIDS prevention, smoking cessation, suicide intervention, substance use prevention, nutrition and weight control, etc., reflecting the social, economic and cultural environment of multiethnic groups in the United States. The PEN-3 model can be described as follows:

1. *Health Education:* In the first phase, the health education planner must be clear on whether the emphasis of the health education curriculum is on the Person, the Extended Family or the Neighborhood (school setting and its surrounding community). A health education program that benefits the entire school system will reach a more diverse audience and promote the concept of "cultural inclusiveness."

2. *Educational Diagnosis of Health Behavior:* In the second phase, the health education planner should explore Perceptions (e.g., knowledge, beliefs, attitudes and behaviors); Enablers (e.g., availability and accessibility of resources, referrals, etc.) and

Nurturers (e.g., reinforcing factors including attitudes and behaviors of health personnel, peers, extended family, kin, employers, religious leaders, media) through the use of surveys or interviews with members of multiethnic groups. It may be appropriate to use nontraditional, less-rigorous data collection methods (e.g., student forums, focus groups, etc.) to ensure consensus and participation.

3. *Cultural Appropriateness of Health Behavior:* Finally, using the information gathered through surveys, interviews, focus groups and other data collection methods, the health education planner should categorize different knowledge, practices, attitudes and beliefs into Positive, Existential and Negative beliefs.

Specifically, positive beliefs and practices are those reinforced by nurturers and enablers that influence members of multiethnic groups attending a school system to engage in health practices that contribute to healthy living. Identified positive health beliefs and practices in a school system should be reinforced and used to empower students and the community.

Existential beliefs and practices are those that have no harmful effect on health status and should not be changed. In this instance, beliefs and practices that may not be understood among other cultures should not be perceived as barriers. Once revealed, existential beliefs and practices can be used to promote positive health beliefs and practices, thus giving students and community residents reassurance that their culture is important and accepted by the school system.

Negative beliefs and practices that place individuals at risk may be influenced by members of the family, the school system or community. Use of negative beliefs and practices is beneficial in designing the intervention; however, both positive and existential beliefs and practices also should be incorporated.

Once all three phases have been completed, it is then necessary to communicate further with identified community leaders and residents who can help determine the most appropriate intervention (health education program) for the school system. Conventional planning efforts in school systems have meant that many ethnic groups feel left out and suspicious. Therefore, members from each ethnic group should participate in initial discussions about health education activities planned for the school system. This process involves not only what health education activities should take place in the school system, but finding ways to involve members from ethnic groups served by the school system in these efforts.

Conclusion

Differences in cultural perspectives often result in misunderstandings between school systems and the ethnic groups served, with no detectable effect on health beliefs and practices (Kumanyika, Morssink and Agurs, 1992). Use of the PEN-3 model can assist health education planners desiring to implement sensitive and appropriate health education curriculums in a multiethnic setting. By using a conceptual approach to identify cultural indices, it becomes less difficult to transfer valuable health information in a manner that is relevant to the lives of students, their families and communities.

References

Airhihenbuwa, C. O. 1990. A conceptual model for cultural appropriate health education programs in developing countries. *International Quarterly of Community Health Education* 11:53-62.

Airhihenbuwa, C. O. 1992. Health promotion and disease prevention strategies for African Americans: A conceptual model. In *Health issues in the Black community*, ed. R. L. Braithwaite and S. E. Taylor, 267-280. San Francisco, CA: Jossey-Bass.

Airhihenbuwa, C. O., R. J. DiClemente, G. Winged and A. Lowe. 1992. HIV/ AIDS education and prevention among African-Americans: A focus on culture. *AIDS Education and Prevention* 4 (3): 207-276.

Airhihenbuwa, C. O., and L. Jack, Jr. 1988. Assessing the level of general well-being among inner-city Black youths. *Journal of Health and Human Resources Administration* 10 (3): 224-241.

Airhihenbuwa, C. O., L. Jack, Jr., and M. Wang. 1991. AIDS knowledge, attitudes and practices among African-American youths. *The Pennsylvania Journal of Physical Education, Health, Recreation and Dance* 61 (3): 18-22.

Airhihenbuwa, C. O., and O. Pineiro. 1988. Cross-cultural health education: A pedagogical challenge. *Journal of School Health* 58 (6): 240-242.

Bailey, E. J. 1987. Sociocultural factors and health care seeking behavior among Black Americans. *Journal of the National Medical Association* 79 (4): 27-31.

Bailey, E. J. 1991. *Urban African-American health care.* Lanham, MD: University Press of America, Inc.

Burney, L., K. Dumars, C. Cheap, H. Nguyen and A. Bustillo. 1989. The impact of cultural variation on the genetic counseling process. *Birth Defects* 23:66-67.

Clark, M. 1959. *Health in the Mexican-American culture.* Berkeley, CA: University of California Press, 47-50.

Communique, S. K., C. Morssink and T. Agurs. 1992. Models for dietary and weight change in African-American women: Identifying cultural components. *Ethnicity and Disease* 12 (2): 166-175.

Diop, C. A. 1991. *Civilization or barbarism: An authentic anthropology.* Brooklyn, NY: Lawrence Hill Books.

Dorfman, S. L. 1990. Health promotion for older minority adults. National Resource Center on Health Promotion and Aging, American Association for Retired Persons, Washington, DC (Publication No. PF4722-991).

Drachman, A. 1992. A stage-of-migration framework for service to immigrant populations. *Social Work* 37 (1): 61-67.

Flaskerud, J. H., and E. Q. Soldevilla. 1986. Filipino and Vietnamese clients: Utilizing an Asian mental health center. *Journal of Psychosocial Nursing* 24:32-36.

Frank-Stromborg, M., and S. J. Olsen. 1993. *Cancer prevention in minority populations: Cultural implications for health care professionals.* Mosby–Year Book, Inc.

Gwaltney, J. L. 1980. *Drylowgso: A self-portrait of Black Americans.* New York: Vintage Books.

Hall, F., and I. E. Harrison. 1993. An observation of university students' perceptual judgments of Black English vs. standard English. Paper Delivered at the National Black Association for Speech-Language and Hearing, Atlanta, Georgia, April 22.

Hannerz, U. 1969. *Soulside.* New York: Columbia University Press.

Harrison, I. E. 1969. *Observations in a Black neighborhood clinic.* Harrisburg, PA: Division of Behavioral Science, Department of Public Health.

Harrison, I. E. 1971. The storefront church as a revitalization movement. In *The Black church in America,* ed. H. Nelson, R. Yorkley, and A. Nelson, 240-245. New York: Basic Books, Inc.

Harrison, I. E. 1975/76. Health status and healing practices: Continuation from an African past. *Journal of African Studies* 2 (4): 554-560.

Harrison, I. E. 1992. Community AIDS education: Trials and tribulations in raising consciousness for prevention. In *African-Americans in the south: Issues of race, class and gender,* ed. H. Baer and Y. Hones, 79-93. Athens, GA: The University of Georgia Press.

Harrison, I. E., and D. S. Harrison. 1971. The Black family experience in health seeking behavior. In *Health and the family: A medical-sociological analysis,* ed. C. O. Crawford, 175-199. New York: Macmillan Company.

Jack, L., Jr. 1988a. Contraceptive knowledge, attitudes and behaviors among Black male adolescents attending a predominately Black university. *Health Education* 19 (3): 22-26.

Jack, L., Jr. 1988b. Sex education: Educating students about themselves. *The Virginia Journal* 11 (1): 16.

Jack, L., Jr., and C. O. Airhihenbuwa. 1992. The impact of selected independent variables on knowledge, attitudes and behaviors among African-American youths. *Wellness Perspective: Research, Theory and Practice* 9:1-4.

Jack, L., Jr., C. O. Airhihenbuwa, F. Murphy, P. Thompson-Reid, B. Wheatley and J. Dickson-Smith.1993. Cancer among low-income African Americans: Implications for culture and community-based health promotion. *Journal of Wellness Perspective: Research, Theory and Practice* 9 (4): 57-68.

Jackson, F. L. C. 1992. Race and ethnicity as biological constructs. *Ethnicity and Disease* 2 (2): 120-125.

Jones, P. H. 1981. *Bad blood: The Tuskegee syphilis experiment.* New York: The Free Press.

Jones, J. M. 1972. *Prejudice and racism.* Reading, MA: Addison-Wesley, 101.

Kemp, C. 1985. Cambodian refugee health care beliefs and practices. *Journal of Community Health Nursing* 2:41-52.

Kumanyika, S. K., C. Morssink and T. Agurs. 1992. Models for dietary and weight change in African-American women: Identifying cultural components. *Ethnicity and Disease* 12 (2): 166-175.

Kunz, K., C. Lam, K. Sui, K. Yeung. 1980. The Chinese. Paper delivered at the Transcultural Health Forum, Honolulu, Hawaii.

Lin-Fu, J. S. 1988. Population characteristics and health care needs of Asian Pacific Americans. *Public Health Reports* 103:18-25.

Locust, C. S. 1985. *Apache beliefs about unwellness and handicaps.* Native American Research and Training Center Monograph Series. Tucson, AZ: University of Arizona.

Locust, C. S. 1987a. *Hopi beliefs about unwellness and handicaps.* Native American Research and Training Center Monograph Series. Tucson, AZ: University of Arizona.

Locust, C. S. 1987b. *Yaqui Indian beliefs about health and handicaps.* Native American Research and Training Center Monograph Series. Tucson, AZ: University of Arizona.

Marín, G. 1991. Research with Hispanic populations. *Applied social research methods series* 23: 28-32.

Martinez, R. 1978. *Hispanic culture and health care.* St. Louis, MO: Mosby.

Paul, B. D. 1955. *Health, culture and community: Case studies of public reactions to health programs.* New York: Russell Sage Foundation.

Radcliffee-Brown, A. R. 1935. On the concept of function in the social sciences. *American Anthropological Association* 37:394-395.

Randall-David, E. 1989. *Strategies for working with culturally diverse communities and clients.* Association for the Care of Children's Health, Bureau of Maternal and Child Health and Resources Development. Publication No. MCH113793. Washington, DC: U.S. Department of Health and Human Services.

Roberson, N. L. 1989. Cancer education programs. In *Minorities and cancer,* ed. L. A. Jones, 107-113. New York: Springer-Verlag.

Smith, E. A. 1993. Cultural and linguistic factors in workers notification to blue collar and non-collar African-Americans. *American Journal of Indian Medicine* 23 (4): 313-335.

Sue, D. W., and D. Sue. 1977. Barriers to effective cross-cultural counseling. *Journal of Counseling Psychology* 24:420-429.

U.S. Department of Health and Human Services. 1985. *Report of the secretary's task force on Black and minority health.* Washington, DC.

Vèlez-Ibàñez, C. G. and Greenberg. 1992. Formation and transformation of funds of knowledge among U.S. Mexican households. *Anthropology and Education Quarterly* 23 (4): 313-335.

Comprehensive Health Education in a Multicultural World

Chapter 4

What Is Comprehensive Health Education?

William M. Kane, PhD, CHES, Lisa Shames, PhD, and Mark Jager, MS

To create schools which provide opportunities for children to reach their fullest health potential requires a collaborative venture among parents, families, communities and school leaders. This chapter provides school leaders with a plan for cooperative planning and implementation of school health programs building on the strengths of multicultural and multiethnic communities. The foundation for planning effective school programs which foster the healthy development of children and youth is constructed of family and community values, strengths and aspirations; community, school and family resources; epidemiologic data; educational and behavioral research (see Figure 1).

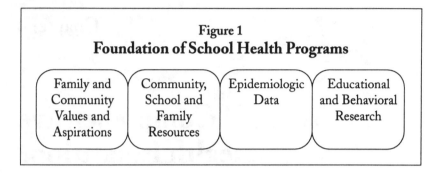

Figure 1
Foundation of School Health Programs

| Family and Community Values and Aspirations | Community, School and Family Resources | Epidemiologic Data | Educational and Behavioral Research |

What Is a Comprehensive School Program to Foster Healthy Development of Children?

The school's role in fostering the healthy development of children and youth goes beyond the teacher providing a health education class. Although health education is a critical component in a child's healthy development, there are other efforts the school should undertake to support the healthy development of children. Allensworth and Kolbe (1987) identified several areas in which schools could establish efforts to promote the health of children, youth and staff. Their framework identifies eight components that can be organized and combined to create a comprehensive program:

- school health education (instruction)
- healthy school environment
- school health services
- physical education/fitness
- nutrition and food services
- school-based counseling and personal support
- schoolsite health promotion
- integrated achool and community health promotion partnerships

This chapter will describe each of these components and provide guidance for school leaders' efforts to provide leadership in organizing the resources of the school and community to promote the healthy development of children and youth. Special attention will be given to development of programs that meet the unique needs of specific cultures and which build on the strengths of multiple cultures.

School Health Education (Instruction)

School health education or instruction is a combination of educational activities with the following aims:
- to increase students' health knowledge
- to develop health-promoting skills
- to provide opportunities for the application of health knowledge and skills
- to reinforce and foster the continued practice of healthy behaviors

Health education is the classroom curricular component of the overall plan to foster healthy development of children and youth. The end goal of school health education is to help individuals acquire the knowledge, skills, opportunities and support to develop to their fullest potential. School health education should be based on a planned and sequential curriculum which interacts with the other components of the comprehensive health education program, families and the community to enable young people to achieve optimal health.

The curriculum is "planned" in that its roots grow from the aspirations of families and communities, the hopes of the students themselves, and the strengths and values of many cultures. It is these foundations upon which school leaders should develop health

curricula. Successful school health education programs are culturally relevant and involve a wide-range of individuals in planning and implementation including:
- students and their families
- community members
- representatives of business, health and social service professions
- clergy
- community activists

Representatives of all these groups should be included in the process of planning a curriculum that is appropriate and sensitive to the cultural needs and values of the community and school. A health education curriculum which builds on the diverse strengths of the community's culture and represents a collectively shared vision of the importance of the health of children is the first step toward helping all children develop to their optimal health potential.

A second "planned" aspect of the school health curriculum is that it should be based on the current documentable threats to the health of children, youth and families. School leaders can look to national, state and local morbidity and mortality statistics for some of this data. Behavioral risk factor data which identifies behaviors that put youth at increased risk of future health problems is also available from the Centers for Disease Control (CDC) and State Departments of Health. In addition, many State Departments of Education are participating in the CDC-sponsored survey which currently collects data regarding risky health behaviors of school-age youth.

Two cautionary notes are in order for school leaders who use population-based morbidity, mortality and risk factor data in planning. These data reports routinely include information on gender, age and race/ethnicity of the population. While such information is helpful in describing those populations who are experiencing disparate health problems, the data should not be used to blame the victims for these health problems. Although alcohol and drug use, smoking, unsafe sexual practices and recklessness are behaviors of individuals, the underlying causes of these behaviors are well rooted in poverty, economics, social class, forced alienation from mainstream society and politics. Large numbers of children of color are born and raised facing these multidimensional stressors. Education should be committed to helping individuals and society resolve these inequalities. Blaming the children, youth and families for risky behaviors and excess morbidity and mortality is an inappropriate role for school leaders and does nothing to improve the health of the community. A second problem with risk factor data is related to sampling techniques used to obtain the data. For example, the CDC sponsored Behavioral Risk Factor Survey utilizes a random digit dialing telephone procedure for collecting data on individual risk factors. Many poor families who are at highest risk do not have telephones. Ethnic/racial minorities are overrepresented in poverty and as a result are undersampled. Similar sampling problems have been noted with the Youth Risk Behavior Survey data. School leaders developing health education programs to serve diverse or multicultural populations should exercise caution when interpreting such data.

Curriculum Content

Although school districts often have different names for the content areas of their particular curricula, the range of topics included in most school health curricula can be grouped into the following ten areas:
- prevention of alcohol and drug use
- nutrition and healthy eating

- family life education
- development of mental and emotional health
- environmental health
- injury prevention and safety
- personal health and healthy exercise and physical fitness
- disease prevention and control
- community health
- selecting health options (consumer health)

All ten content areas are not covered at each grade level. Decisions regarding scope and focus of the curriculum at each grade level are based on what is appropriate to community interests and needs, and physical and mental development of students. The health education curriculum and content should be sequential, each year building on and reinforcing the knowledge learned and the skills developed at earlier grade levels. A basic principle is that students should acquire knowledge and skills prior to their exposure to the opportunities where they need to apply such knowledge and skills. For example, if children in your community are faced with opportunities and pressure to experiment with tobacco use at age 10, they need to have specific knowledge and skills to resist pressure to engage in tobacco use prior to age 10. The importance of a health education curriculum built on specific community values and needs becomes obvious.

Health Skills
Health education curricula include both content and process. The process, or *skills development*, is a major focus of the curriculum and classroom activities. These health-related skills are defined a bit differently by each school district, but fall into the following general categories.

- assessing personal health and risks
- gathering and assessing health information
- rewarding healthy behavior
- communicating with others
- making decisions
- negotiating for health
- managing stress
- setting and achieving goals

School leaders will want to develop a curriculum which provides learning opportunities for students to acquire an awareness of and knowledge regarding health; skills and opportunities to practice healthy behavior; and encouragement and reinforcement for developing healthy lifestyles. A curriculum of this type relies heavily on experiential learning.

Unlike curricula in many areas, a health curriculum is constantly in a state of change, reflecting developments in culture, society, technology and behavioral sciences. An annual review should be conducted to determine the relevance of the curriculum to the changing or evolving priorities and needs of the local community.

Instructional Time

Planning for instructional time is another important issue school leaders will want to consider in developing the school health education program. Most authorities recommend that elementary and middle school students experience the equivalent of two to three hours of health education each week. Integration of health education learning experiences into other subject-oriented learning experiences can be successfully accomplished.

However, experience shows that many schools which report using the integrated approach are not successful in helping students gain the knowledge, develop the skills and provide the opportunities to practice healthy behaviors. This lack of success may be due not to the integrated approach, but to the level of commitment, time and priority the teachers and school place on quality health instruction. Many leaders recommend that elementary schools establish specific times for health instruction as well as integrate health education into other subjects in the curriculum.

Health education should continue beyond elementary school. Early adolescence is a critical time; young people are exploring various behaviors, making choices and establishing lifetime health behaviors. Health education in grades seven and eight should include 60 to 70 hours of direct instruction and learning experiences each year. At the high school level students should be encouraged to include at least two semesters of health instruction in their schedules.

Teacher Skills and Preparation

The skill and preparation of the classroom teacher is critical to the success of school health education. Teachers should be professionally prepared, either through preservice or inservice education, to implement the health curriculum, to foster health-related learning, to help students develop health and life skills, and to work with the school, families and communities to provide opportunities to practice this healthy behavior.

Teachers should keep in mind that the health needs and interests of their students will be personal and will differ from student to student, from class to class and from community to community. The optimal school health education program will allow the skilled teacher to modify learning opportunities accordingly.

Teachers should be fully prepared in the following areas:
- handling controversial health issues and content
- experiential learning

- peer education, cooperative learning and cross-tutoring
- questioning strategies to foster development of critical thinking
- health counseling
- family relations and counseling
- advocacy
- life skills training
- rewarding healthy behavior
- modeling healthy behavior

Administrative Leadership

Administrative leadership in providing policy, funding and support for training and materials to implement successful health education programs is also important. School leaders have a responsibility to work with communities, initiating action and providing leadership in policy and funding areas. Effective school programs have their roots in the community. Administrative leadership involves working with communities to facilitate program development in order to establish relevant health education programs.

Instructional Materials

Instructional and educational materials for health instruction include a wide range of textbooks, pre-packaged curricula and supplementary texts, videos and materials which can be used in conjunction with local and state developed curricula or commercial curricula.

Healthy School Environment

A safe and healthful environment is important for education. School should be a place where students and teachers do not fear for their personal safety. Harassment from gang members and drug pushers and resolution of conflict by violent actions have no place in the school.

Commitment to providing a safe environment, regular safety inspections, emergency drills, safe and orderly transportation, adherence to environmental regulations and standards, and clean, safe and well-maintained school grounds and buildings communicates a message to all by establishing health norms and expectations. The physical surroundings in which students and teachers are expected to work should promote healthful behaviors.

Likewise, students' personal achievement and social growth is fostered by the psychological environment of the school. Teachers serve as health role models for their students. The emotional and physical health and the social, problem solving and conflict-management skills demonstrated by teachers influence young people.

Not surprisingly research has found that among the frequently encountered positive role models in the lives of children is a favorite teacher. Teachers are not only developers of academic skills, but also positive models for students' personal identification and development. It is critical that all children and youth have teacher role models with whom they can identify. Selection and professional development of teachers representing the cultural diversity of the community is an important consideration.

The health norms and social expectations created by the school act as factors to support healthy development of students. Benard (1991) has identified the level of caring and support within the school as a powerful predictor of positive outcomes for youth.

Researchers have concluded that schools which are successful in helping young people overcome problem behaviors project clear expectations and regulations, emphasize academics, have high levels of student participation, foster high self-esteem, and promote social and scholastic success. Schools that establish high expectations for all students and provide them the support necessary to achieve them have high rates of academic success. It is critical that healthy expectations derive from and are consistent with community cultural values.

Benard's review of the research on the school's role in developing resilient youth concludes that the caregiving environment of the school serves as a protective shield in reducing levels of alcohol and drug use.

School Health Services

The provision of health services by schools emerged near the end of the nineteenth century in response to compulsory education laws. The focus of these services was to prevent and control infectious diseases and exclude those children who represented a health threat to others.

Much has changed over the past 100 years. The 1990 Joint Commission on Health Education Terminology definition of school health services identified both the school health services personnel and their responsibilities. School health service personnel include the following individuals that serve to appraise, protect, and promote the health of students and school personnel.

- physicians
- nurses
- dentists
- health educators
- allied health personnel
- social workers
- teachers

That definition goes on to describe school health services as those activities designed to:

- ensure access to and appropriate use of primary health care services
- prevent and control communicable disease
- provide emergency care for injury or sudden illness
- promote and provide optimum sanitary conditions in a safe school facility and environment
- provide concurrent learning opportunities which are conducive to the maintenance and promotion of individual and community health

For example, health services provided by the school and community to all students in one Massachusetts school district include:

- immunizations
- vision and hearing screening
- fluoride dental rinse program
- dental screening, sealants and cavity repair
- physical evaluation
- speech therapy
- postural screening
- pediculosis (body lice) screening
- health assessment and individual education plans
- child abuse assessments
- prekindergarten and kindergarten screening
- management of asthmatics
- mental health counseling and referral
- family outreach/parent support groups
- inservice education for staff
- supplemental health education in classrooms

School nurses have traditionally been the focal point for health services in the schools. In addition, school nurses are a key resource for the other components of the overall school health program by providing health education and acting as consultants on community and family health.

Unfortunately there are only about 30,000 school nurses throughout the country to serve 42 million students. The National School Nurses Association recommends a ratio of one nurse for every 750 students. To achieve this ratio, we would need more than twenty thousand additional school nurses. In the absence of adequate funding for school nurses, many schools rely on a school secretary to administer first aid and minor medications.

As a result of rapidly escalating costs of health care combined with today's unstable market for employment, many adults and their children have no medical insurance and limited access to primary health care. As a result many schools (and communities) are exploring alternative methods of providing health services for young people.

More than 100 health clinics based in schools have emerged over the past decade. These clinics provide a full range of primary health care services and act as a point of referral for students requiring more extensive diagnostic work, treatment and rehabilitation.

Unfortunately many of these clinics have become embroiled in controversy surrounding the provision of sexuality counseling and birth control devices. By the end of high school, 60.8 percent of males and 48 percent of females report they have had sexual intercourse (U.S. Department of Health and Human Services, 1991). About 60,000 babies are born each year to adolescent girls under 15 years of age. Family planning counseling and provision of services are appropriate roles for school-based clinics.

Some schools (and communities) are experimenting with health insurance coverage for students. Actually, the concept of "accident" insurance for students has been around for decades. Today's student health insurance has been expanded to cover regular check-ups, immunizations, hospitalizations, outpatient care, prescriptions, eye glasses, and drug and alcohol treatment and rehabilitation. These insurance plans are being financed through community fundraising, public health agencies, and private insurance carriers.

In every school the physical and mental health needs of some students will exceed the immediate resources of the school and its personnel. Paying for health care is an expensive and complex societal issue. However, good health is essential for learning and achieving one's fullest potential. School leaders need to work closely with families, community leaders, and health and social service providers to establish a systematic health care system for students.

Physical Education/Fitness

It is widely held that participation in physical education activities promotes health development. More than 97 percent of this country's elementary school children and 80 percent of its secondary school students have access to organized physical education.

Students in elementary schools participate in physical education an average of 3.1 times weekly, with 36.4 percent taking classes daily. At the high school level, students engage in physical education an average of 3.9 times weekly, with 36.3 percent taking classes daily (Office of Disease Prevention and Health Promotion, 1984).

The popular literature attributes a large range of benefits to physical exercise, including:

- improved cardiovascular and physiological functioning
- reduction of stress
- reduction of weight and body fat
- improved skeletal and muscle structure
- increased sense of self-worth
- improved academic performance

Indeed, research findings seem to support many of these popular beliefs. Yet despite the growing body of knowledge regarding the effects of physical fitness and exercise on health and the long existence of physical education programs in America's schools, all is not well. The National Children and Youth Fitness Study released in 1984 cited the following problems:

- Body fat of today's youth is significantly greater than in the 1960s.
- Only 50 percent of today's youth participate in appropriate physical activity.
- Only 50 percent of the students in twelfth grade participate in physical education classes.
- Physical education teachers devote most classroom time to competitive sports and other activities that have questionable health effects and that cannot readily be performed once one reaches adulthood.

Recognizing the importance of exercise the U.S. Department of Health and Human Services *Healthy People 2000* recommends that by the year 2000 "schools increase by at least 50 percent (from 36 percent to 54 percent) the proportion of children and adolescents in 1st through 12th grade who participate in daily school physical education" (Objective #1.8).

The proportion of students participating in daily physical education is one measure of the quality of school-based physical education. Other measures of quality identified by *Healthy People 2000* are students' exposure to information about how and why to participate in activities and encouragement to develop skills that allow for out-of-school and lifetime activities. Lifetime physical activities are defined as those activities in which an individual can participate throughout his or her life. These include tennis, badminton, golf, hiking, individual exercise, swimming and bicycling. They do not include football, soccer, baseball, basketball or most competitive team activities that commonly dominate the high school curriculum.

Healthy People 2000 recommends that by the year 2000 we "Increase to at least 50 percent (baseline 27 percent in 1984) the proportion of school physical education class time that students spend being physically active, preferably engaged in lifetime physical activities" (Objective #1.9). Studies indicate that only 27 percent of the current physical education classroom time is spent in actual physical activity; while 26 percent is spent in instruction, 22 percent is spent in administrative tasks and 25 percent is spent waiting.

Physical education is another area of the school health program which requires coordination between schools, families and communities. The typical student in fifth through twelfth grades reports that more than 80 percent of his or her physical activity takes place outside of physical education classes. The majority of this time is spent in activities sponsored by community organizations, including religious groups, parks and recreation programs, local teams and private organizations.

Healthy People 2000 calls for more class time to be spent engaged in lifetime activities and more emphasis given to developing knowledge, attitudes, cognitive skills and physical skills students need to remain physically active throughout life.

In order to achieve these objectives and provide physical education experiences which promote the healthy development of students, teachers responsible for these program need preservice or inservice education. District or school level physical education specialists can become responsible for the inservice education of nonspecialized teachers responsible for physical education classes. In addition, a team including the physical education specialist should assume responsibility for overall curriculum scope, sequence and implementation.

Nutrition and Food Services

The history of school nutrition in America is a study in politics. The establishment of school lunch programs in America coincided with America's overproduction of food. School lunches became a convenient "dumping ground" for surplus food commodities which in turn provided low-cost food for America's children. Surplus farm products (milk, eggs, meat, cheese) were not always the healthiest foods.

At the same time, nutrition education emerged as an important function of the U.S. Department of Agriculture, the same organization that had encouraged overproduction of food and established the school lunch assistance programs. In the late 1970s the U.S. Department of Health and Human Services, after long and difficult negotiations with the Department of Agriculture, made a series of recommendations in *Dietary Guidelines for Americans*. Those recommendations urged Americans to:

- reduce intake of fat to less than 30 percent and saturated fats to less than 10 percent of the total dietary intake
- increase consumption of fruits and vegetables
- reduce intake of sugar
- increase consumption of whole grain products
- reduce consumption of salt
- reduce total calorie intake

These guidelines established new criteria for measuring the nutritional value of school lunch programs. Although many schools today incorporate the principle of the *Dietary Guidelines,* such nutritional planning should be universal.

Healthy People 2000 recommends we "increase to at least 90 percent the proportion of school lunch and breakfast services... that are consistent with the nutritional principles in the *Dietary Guidelines for Americans*" (Objective #2.17). To accomplish this objective, school meals must provide choices that include low-fat foods, vegetables, fruits and whole-grain products. Doing so will also provide opportunities for students to practice the health knowledge and food selection skills introduced in school-based health education instruction.

To support this learning experience, *Healthy People 2000* recommends that schools offer "point-of-choice" nutrition information in the school cafeteria. Point-of-choice nutrition information includes information on nutrient value and calories of the foods being served. Such information enables students to choose healthy food.

Healthy People 2000 further recommends that school fundraising activities that involve food sales, on-site vending machine offerings and food service offerings at concession stands during recreational and other events should also reflect the principles of the *Dietary Guidelines for Americans.*

For many children, especially poor children, school breakfast, lunch and snack programs constitute a significant portion of their daily nutritional intake. In these cases, school food service personnel, and particularly cafeteria managers are the gatekeepers to school children's food supply. The school's nutritional program provides an excellent opportunity to establish health norms and model healthy nutritional behaviors. Schools which provide healthy food choices and discourage availability of unhealthy foods send a clear message to developing youth. Schools can also involve students in the planning of menus and preparation of food as a hands-on learning experience.

School-based nutritional offerings that are both healthy and culturally appropriate for the community are important considerations. Providing opportunities for children and youth to establish food selection and eating patterns which are not available in or consistent with the community values, will have little chance of becoming lifetime health behaviors. Careful thought and planning should precede the establishment of culturally appropriate and healthy school meals.

Nutritional policies consistent with scientific health findings and the best interest of students demonstrate a school's commitment to the development of healthy youth. Such policies with opportunities for students to practice nutritional knowledge and food selection skills in the lunch line, are consistent with the overall concept of a healthy school.

In some communities school food service personnel spend time in the classroom working with teachers delivering nutrition instruction to students and preparing educational materials which enable students' families to support the classroom instruction. For students with special nutritional needs close cooperation between school health services personnel and food services personnel is a critical factor in the students' achievement of optimal health.

School-Based Counseling and Personal Support

The school counseling program was originally implemented in the 1960s to provide vocational guidance for students. Today school counselors and psychologists work in partnership with teachers, parents and community personnel to respond to special needs and provide personal support for individual students, teachers and staff. In addition, in many schools counseling staff have initiated programs which promote schoolwide mental, emotional and social well-being.

The American School Counselor Association (ASCA) identifies the major aims of school-based counseling as follows:

- to help students increase communication skills
- improve the quality of interaction between adults and youth
- to encourage the learning process
- to sensitize administrators and teachers to the necessity of matching the curriculum to the developmental needs of the students

The school counselor works to meet these goals by "structuring developmental guidance to promote psychological aspects of human development; individual and small group counseling; consultation with and inservice training for staff, parents and community groups; and performing needs assessments to guide interventions" (Klingman, 1984).

A recent study found that school counselors routinely interacted with students on the following issues:

- divorce
- substance abuse by students or their parents
- teen sexuality and pregnancy
- depression
- suicide
- sexual and physical abuse
- problems with family members or friends
- concerns about career and future
- questions about the meaning of life

Counselors also often become involved in providing assistance to teachers and other school staff and their families. The activities of school counselors often bring them into contact with families of students and with community health and social service workers. Counselors often become advocates for students' interests.

Like teachers, counselors must be sensitive to the unique cultural backgrounds of the students and their families. An understanding of the family and cultural values which guide students' priorities and decisions is critical for all who are responsible for helping young people grow up healthy. Schools should make special efforts to select and prepare counselors who have background and understanding of the communities and cultures in which students live.

Counselors can provide broad-based intervention programs to promote the health of students. They can initiate individual and small group programs aimed at preventing the onset of mental and emotional health problems, as well as interventions designed to reduce the consequences of stress or rehabilitate those who are experiencing difficulty in coping with the stresses of life. These interventions include:

- problem-solving training
- assertiveness training
- life skills training
- peer led problem solving groups
- programs to build self-esteem and address loss of control, peer pressure and adolescent rebellion (Klingman, 1984).

Many schools employ school psychologists. The role of the psychologist varies from school to school. Much of the school psychologist's time is spent on pyschoeducational evaluation and educational programming for students with special needs. In addition, the school psychologist provides:

- group appraisal of students
- coordination with other pupil personnel workers
- coordination with child and youth-serving community agencies
- counseling and psychotherapy
- preventive mental health consultation
- participation on curriculum committees
- inservice education
- data collection and research.

School counselors and psychologists are important members of the team who contribute to the healthy development of students. Both the counselor and psychologist play an important role in linking schools with families and community health and social service workers and agencies. These resulting partnerships are crucial to creating an environment that supports young people in growing up healthy.

Schoolsite Health Promotion

Health promotion is a combination of educational, organizational and environmental activities designed to encourage school students and staff to adopt healthier lifestyles and become better consumers of health care services (Comprehensive Health Education Resources Center, 1989). Like all components in a comprehensive school health program, school-based health promotion is intertwined and closely linked to the other components.

School leaders should view health promotion as a systems approach which enables the school to bring together the various health-related components to foster a culture which supports healthful development and the practice of healthy lifestyles. Health promotion establishes the social climate with the following characteristics:

- Teachers and family members are encouraged to model healthful behavior.
- Opportunities are provided for students, faculty and staff, and parents and community members to practice health promoting behaviors.
- Reinforcement is built-in through recognizing and rewarding those who practice healthy behaviors.
- Health services are linked to health instruction.
- Assessment, counseling and, when necessary, referral of students experiencing health-related problems are provided.
- School policies and administrative procedures consistently support the healthful development of youth, teachers and staff.

The documented effects of health promotion programs on staff include increase in energy level, increased productivity, improved morale, decreased absenteeism and decreased teacher burnout.

Teachers and school staff who model health knowledge, skills and behaviors learned by students in the classroom encourage students to adopt healthful behaviors. School policies and practices that provide a health promoting environment free from violence and pressures to engage in self-destructive health behaviors provide an opportunity for the students to adopt those healthful behaviors.

Providing for the safety of students is only the first step in establishing a health promoting environment in the school. Schools can provide other health promoting opportunities as well. These include:

- opportunities to select food in the school cafeteria which is low in fat, high in nutrients and prepared in a healthy manner

- a smoke-free environment in which to learn
- opportunities for all students to engage in physical activities which promote cardiovascular fitness, flexibility, strength, co-ordination and that can be practiced over the life span.

Social values and cultural beliefs and traditions are important determinants of health behavior. The school must reach beyond the schoolyard gate and work with families and communities to understand the cultural aspects of health. Then it can help communities and families develop culturally specific programs which enable them to provide health promoting activities that reinforce those of the school.

The health and social norms of the home and community support or detract from a school's ability to foster the development of healthy youth. Communities that value healthful behavior can send a clear message supporting young people's adoption of healthy behaviors. The following activities can be part of that message:

- modeling healthy behavior
- providing environmental support (such as enforcement of laws against the sale of alcohol to minors)
- having health care providers inquire about and offer counseling regarding healthy behaviors
- providing opportunities for young and old alike to practice health promoting behavior

The school's role in establishing the health promotion component includes:

- appointment of a "leader"
- formation of a school and community health council
- work with the community and families to conceive and articulate a vision for the healthy development of children
- analysis of the current school, community and family environ-

ment for promoting health and supporting the healthy development of students

- development and implementation of new policies, programs and strategies that fully utilize the resources of the school, community and families to help children grow up healthy

As with all programs, education and training will enhance the success of the school health promotion program. In more than one half of the states, department of education and department of health leaders offer five-day statewide summer wellness conferences for school teams comprised of administrators, teachers, staff and community leaders.

These teams learn how to incorporate the concept of "wellness as a lifestyle" into their personal and professional lives. When these teams return to their home communities, they have knowledge, skills and commitment to establish health promotion efforts in their schools and communities.

Integrated School and Community Health Promotion Partnerships

Smoking, alcohol and drug abuse, sexual activity at an early age, violence and abuse, delinquency and school drop out are not only school problems. These threats to the future health of youth are interrelated. They share common roots in the community, family and school.

Partnerships to unite schools, families and communities are being established across America to help solve these community-wide problems. These effective collaborative partnerships focus on health promotion and disease prevention. They are the cornerstone of prevention and the foundation upon which children develop to their fullest potential. School officials have a leadership role to play in these collaborative efforts.

Schools and communities cannot ignore the role poverty plays in limiting children's access to health and education and subsequently, the opportunities for success in the twenty-first century. Appropriate health education for poor children and children of diverse ethnic backgrounds should be devised in consultation with those who represent their cultures. Partnerships formed to support healthy development of children must involve parents from all cultures, business and community leaders representing the diversity of the community, and parents and members of poor communities. To ignore this area will result in social and educational failure for millions of young people. For many, this failure will be a precursor of an adult life of poor health, crime, unemployment, welfare dependency and premature death. This is an unacceptable vision for our children. Coalitions and partnerships driven by mutual aspirations sharing a common vision of healthy young people can effectively help schools meet the needs of youth.

Code Blue: Uniting for Healthier Youth—A Call to Action, a report of the National Commission on the Role of the School and Community in Improving Adolescent Health (1990), issued a call for national action to improve the health of youth. The Commission was jointly convened by the National Association of State Boards of Education and the American Medical Association. This report identified all sectors of society including:

- individual Americans
- federal and state governments
- local communities
- health and social services communities
- businesses and corporations
- media, entertainment and advertising industries
- churches, youth-serving agencies and other community organizations
- the education community

Recommendations for collaborative action were directed to each of these sectors. Among those recommendations aimed at the education community were the following:

- Education and health are inextricably intertwined and achieving their education mission will require attending to the health needs of students.
- Recognize the necessity of working with not only [students], but their families, whatever the composition of that family might be.
- Promote the concept of collaboration within the school and welcome other health professionals and service delivery organizations to the school as full partners in working with students.
- Permit sharing of information with collaborating agencies on a need-to-know basis that maintains confidentiality.
- Allow schools to serve as locations for [student] health care if the local community determines that school sites are the most effective location for providing collaborative services.
- Make school buildings available as sites for recreation, services, and other community activities outside school hours.
- Provide all students opportunities to engage in community service.

The Commission concluded the recommendations to the education community by urging education leaders to assure that teachers are trained in collaborative approaches and provided sufficient time to work with other professionals, community members and families.

Collaboration with families requires that schools engage these families in the education of their children. This can be done by giving families meaningful roles in school governance, communicating with families about the school program and student progress, and offering families opportunities to support the learning process at home and at school (Carnegie Council on Adolescent Development, 1989). For example, homework assignments which draw on their families' history and experiences, or the views regarding current health affairs serve to engage youth and their families with the school.

References

Allensworth, D. D., and L. J. Kolbe. 1987. The comprehensive school health program: Exploring an expanded concept. *Journal of School Health* 57 (10): 409-412.

American School Health Association, Association for the Advancement of Health Education and Society for Public Health Education. 1989. *National adolescent student health survey.* Oakland, CA: Third Party Press.

Benard, B. 1991. Fostering resiliency in kids: Protective factors in the family, school and community. *Western Regional Center for Drug-Free Schools and Communities.* Portland, OR: NWREL.

Carnegie Council on Adolescent Development, Task Force on Education of Young Adolescents. 1989. *Turning points: Preparing American youth for the 21st century.* Washington, DC.

Kane, W. M. 1993. *Step by step to comprehensive school health: The program planning guide.* Santa Cruz, CA: ETR Associates.

Klingman, A. 1984. Health-related school guidance: Practical application in primary prevention. *Personnel and Guidance Journal* 62:576-579.

National Commission on the Role of the School and the Community in Improving Adolescent Health. 1990. *Code blue: Uniting for healthier youth.* Alexandria, VA: National Association of State Boards of Education.

Office of Disease Prevention and Health Promotion. 1984. *Key findings: National children and youth fitness study II.* Washington, DC.

U.S. Department of Agriculture and U.S. Department of Health and Human Services. 1990. *Nutrition and your health: Dietary guidelines for Americans.* 3d ed. Home and Garden Bulletin No. 232. Washington, DC.

U.S. Department of Health and Human Services, Public Health Service. 1991. *Healthy people 2000: National health promotion and disease prevention objectives.* DHHS Publication No. (PHS) 95-50212. Washington, DC.

Chapter 5

A Multiethnic Perspective on Comprehensive Health Education

Anthony R. Sancho, PhD

Comprehensive health education in the United States has been a manifestation of "mainstream" American values toward health issues and behaviors. Embedded in this has been a strong puritanical ethic that has allowed little room for diversity of values and beliefs about health and wellness among the many ethnic groups that make up America. Considerable discussion has occurred about what comprehensive health education is and the debate continues. This chapter does not attempt to argue for a definition of health education, but rather focuses on issues that must be addressed in developing and delivering comprehensive health education to multiethnic/multilingual populations in the context of American society. The assumption here is that most health education programs need to become more sensitive to the growing diversity in this country.

Schools have been given initiatives to deal with issues of health, health education, substance abuse, HIV education, as well as a variety of other tasks addressing social issues above and beyond the core curriculum. Yet most administrators and teachers have had little, if any, formal training in dealing with these social phenomena. To compound the issue, most educators have little or no knowledge of the beliefs and attitudes of the many cultural groups that make up the American tapestry. Therefore, cultural clash is an everyday occurrence in our schools.

To address some key issues associated with a multiethnic perspective on comprehensive health education, three questions will be posed:

1. How can we make comprehensive health education relevant to multiethnic/multilingual students?

2. What are some of the challenges and opportunities in delivering comprehensive health education to multiethnic student populations?

3. What should a multiethnic/multilingual health education program look like?

Making Comprehensive Health Education Relevant

In response to the first question—How can we make comprehensive health education relevant to multiethnic/multilingual students?—it is absolutely necessary to develop an awareness of students' cultural, social, economic and political roots in order to have a positive influence on the way health education is structured. Equally important is gaining knowledge of the students' family values and traditions. Another key element is having an understanding of students' and families' degrees of acculturation into mainstream American values and behaviors. It is important to note that the process of acculturation is a continuum along which a given individual moves throughout his/her life, not a static position permanently maintained. These degrees range from recent immigrants who cling to the values and traditions of their native country to those racial and ethnic groups that have been in America for generations and are fully acculturated. However, individuals acculturate more quickly in some areas of their lives than in others. For example, some students may be more acculturated in the areas of food and dress, while remaining traditional in the areas of religion and language.

While culture plays an important role in shaping individuals, students have unique personalities and histories within their cultures. Effective teachers regard each student as an individual, with personal preferences, strengths and weaknesses, family background, and history. Caution should be taken not to lump students and families from a particular ethnic group into one category. Even though there will be some similarities within a group, many differences will also exist among its members.

To make comprehensive health education more relevant to the diverse groups in American schools, teachers and administrators must gain a better understanding of these students. Information related to the following sample questions can be obtained from students and their families through classroom activities and observations. Use caution in asking direct questions that may intrude on privacy.

- What is the country of origin of your students' families?
- Are they immigrants?
- Have they lived in the community for a long time?
- Do they retain family ties in their mother country?
- What language is spoken at home?
- What foods do they like to eat?
- What holidays or other traditions do they celebrate at home?
- Where do they seek health care?
- What do they want to be when they grow up?

- Who is in their families? Who of these live in the same house?
- How is authority distributed among family members?
- What are the rights and responsibilities of each family member?
- What are the attitudes, expectations, and behaviors toward individuals at different stages in the life cycle?
- What behaviors at home are appropriate or unacceptable for the students?
- How is the behavior of children/youth traditionally controlled?
- What range of behaviors are considered "work" and what range are considered "play"?

To answer these or similar questions, discussions with students may be held in small groups or as a total class, although caution should be used with direct questioning. A simple activity such as placing pins on a map of the world to show what country each student or the student's family is from, can show the diversity in the classroom. If students are shy, ask them to respond to questions on paper or index cards. These are just a few examples of ways to gain a better understanding of the students and their home life.

Learn about the students' environment. Drive around the students' neighborhoods to become familiar with their resources and their contextual environment. Find out where they shop, which health clinics they use, and which community recreation areas are available in the community. Are there many billboards advertising alcohol and tobacco? How many liquor stores and fast-food restaurants are there? Where do youth tend to congregate? Read the local newspaper to keep up with local issues. Pay attention to the strengths of the community and what positive actions people are taking. Talk to the school nurse and/or counselor to learn the most common health issues among the students. Talk to public health personnel at clinics and hospitals about the community's health issues.

Another means of making health education more relevant to multiethnic populations is to ask individual students and their families what their concerns are about health and what they want to learn about health. Health education focuses on the development of healthy lifestyles. Teaching will not be successful if it tries to force all students to adopt one specific lifestyle. Data suggest that health messages are more readily accepted if they do not conflict with existing cultural beliefs. Where appropriate, messages should acknowledge existing cultural values and practices, building on cultural strengths and pride. Several cultural factors, such as family values, religious beliefs, health beliefs, and communication styles, affect health education instruction and how it is accepted and internalized by students and their families.

Challenges and Opportunities

In addressing the second question—What are some of the challenges and opportunities in delivering comprehensive health education to multiethnic student populations?—educators will have to adapt and/or develop health curricula that are meaningful and sensitive to the backgrounds of their students. Even though health is a universal concern, the way health care is accessed and the development of healthy lifestyles are predisposed by group and individual beliefs and experiences. The major challenges to the health educator revolve around having a thorough understanding and knowledge of the clients' perceptions and attitudes as they relate to the following issues.

Family Values

The family is a very strong and influential institution in all cultures. However, the definition of family and how it is manifested varies from group to group. In some cultures the family includes the extended family, such as neighbors, godparents, aunts and uncles, second and third cousins, and close friends. Also, some families are extremely group-oriented, even in decision making. All members may have a say in adopting family rules and solving family problems, including health-related concerns. For example, many Hispanic/Latino families share the common bond, *cariño*, a very deep sense of unqualified care and protection. Family members are considered equal and unconditionally accepted; they are valued simply because they exist, not because of what they have done or not done. For most Latinos, revealing secrets and looking for answers outside the family unit go against their culture. The Hispanic family tends to give financial and emotional support to all its members. They care for the old and infirm, take care of and protect the children of the extended family, and give a sense of belonging to all members.

In most multiethnic cultures, the strength of the family aids in coping with the stress that often results from conflicts between mainstream American culture and minority cultures. Such conflicts, usually involving parents and children, may arise from negative messages they receive about their cultures, such as racism, low income, unemployment, poor school performance, peer value differences, and acculturation or adjustment to American culture. The family counteracts these negative messages to protect its members.

Gender and role differences also play a significant part in how various cultures perceive family relationships. These perceptions affect how health care is accessed and how family members interact with one another during times of crisis or illness. Again, this varies considerably according to the degree of acculturation.

Linguistic Diversity

In 1990, more than 31.8 million people—14 percent of the U.S. population aged 5 or over—indicated they spoke a language other than English in the home. Spanish is the most common non-English language spoken in the United States with 17,399,172 speakers, representing 54 percent of the language-minority population. Four other language groups have more than one million speakers: French, German, Italian, and Chinese. In addition, immigration of non-English-speaking Southeast Asians continues. In 1992, the Census Bureau released data on the school-age population of non-English speakers (ages 5–17), reporting that 6.3 million children, or 14 percent of the total school-age population do not speak English at home. This represents a 38 percent increase over the past ten years.

This increasing linguistic diversity has tremendous implications for the structuring and delivery of health education instruction. For language-minority youngsters, a bilingual mode would be the most appropriate method; however, most health educators are not bilingual and there are few health education materials available in languages other than English. Therefore, other methodologies need to be employed to make health education concepts comprehensible to speakers of other languages. One such method is "Sheltered English Instruction," which is discussed in detail in another chapter in this book.

Religious Beliefs

Religion plays a significant role in how multiethnic groups view health and well-being. Both Christian and non-Christian sects have extremely diverse beliefs as they relate to the influences that their deities have on wellness and physical, as well as spiritual life. Among many groups, religious beliefs play a part in their daily lives, particularly when dealing with illness and physical well-being. Nontraditional religious beliefs can also come into play. More traditional Latinos, for example, maintain nontraditional beliefs that draw heavily from the teachings of the Catholic church, mixing the belief in God and the saints with psychic powers and the spiritual work of folk healers. Health educators need to be sensitive to these beliefs and tailor the health education curriculum so as not to alienate cultural groups who have maintained these beliefs and traditions for generations. In meeting this challenge, educators should consult priests, ministers, and community leaders to learn of a particular group's religious beliefs toward health and wellness.

Health Beliefs

For many multiethnic populations, illness traditionally has its roots in physical imbalances or supernatural forces. God's will, magical powers, or evil spirits often are assumed to have caused an illness. Often, no differentiation is made between physical and emotional illness. Many groups seek alternative methods of health care, often consulting folk healers, using home remedies, herbs, and other adjunctive therapies. Lower socioeconomic status and lack of health insurance may significantly influence attitudes about health and access to health care.

Communication Styles

Communication styles are predisposed by culture, socioeconomic status, levels of educational achievement, and language. Different groups also have different ways of expressing emotions and feelings, from physical interaction to verbal tone. With many groups, delicate subjects associated with health issues such as sex, drug abuse, cleanliness, etc. are frequently not discussed. Most multiethnic groups are hesitant to disclose personal or family information to a stranger and are not open to group counseling or therapy.

If school communication with students and parents must be done in a language other than English, caution should be taken in translating materials. Often, direct word-for-word translations do not convey the same meaning or concept and can create miscommunication or misunderstanding. Therefore, persons literate in these other languages should do the translations and should have an understanding of the literacy levels of the target audiences.

Opportunities for Delivering Health Education

In these days of intense debate over health care and educational reform, schools are under tremendous pressure to address educational and health issues and to provide more effective instruction to their students. The challenges are great, but the opportunity for comprehensive health education to be a major unifying force in school reform is exciting. The following list contains only some of the opportunities that health education can provide.

* Health education is a content area that is cross-curricular. Its subject matter can form the basis for units in language arts, reading, math, science, social studies, and of course, physical education.
* Health education topics lend themselves well to bringing parents and the community into closer ties with the school.
* By infusing a multiethnic perspective into health education, both students and parents can develop a greater awareness and understanding of other cultural groups, thus lessening racism and racial conflicts which are so visible on school campuses today.
* Through a multiethnic perspective administrators, school boards, and school staffs will begin to develop a greater sensitivity towards the growing number of diverse populations in the United States.
* A multiethnic/multilingual perspective on health education

could serve to encourage both students and school staff to appreciate multiculturalism and bilingualism as positive forces in preparing for life in the twenty-first century.

• Health education can promote partnerships between schools, public agencies, the private sector, community groups, and youth groups.

Multiethnic/Multilingual Health Education

In addressing the third question—What should a multiethnic/multilingual health education program look like?—one needs to look at the current status and content of comprehensive health education in America. Most health curricula are based on the following units of study: Community/Environmental Health, Consumer Health, Disease Prevention and Control, Substance Abuse Prevention, Family Life, Physical Fitness, Safety, Growth and Development, and Nutrition. A close review of the content of the most popular programs in this country reveals that little or no attention is paid to the beliefs and values of diverse populations. A few are beginning to utilize translations, and some display other than White persons in their graphics, but the content is still primarily based on middle class mainstream American values. It is obvious that this failure to address the diversity of peoples in this nation weakens the effectiveness of health education, and, in some cases, even adds to the conflict between cultures.

Health educators, administrators, school board members, and curriculum developers must appreciate diversity in a sincere and sensitive way, not just pay lip service to it. This calls for developing a strong and viable partnership with the community. Delivering health instruction in a language that is understandable to students and their families is critical. Materials must reflect all the groups represented in the school and the community. A comprehensive staff development program in multicultural awareness and ethnic pluralism should be implemented. Health education should be infused into all areas of the curriculum.

An ideal health education program is one that is student-centered. The student should be at the center of what is taught, using their and their parents' areas of interest and concerns about health and wellness. The languages and cultures of *all* students need to be taken into account in planning and adapting the curriculum. At the same time it is important to not neglect the cultures and background of mainstream students. They too have a culture. Even though the melting pot theory has prevailed in America since this nation was established, all students need to be made aware that at some point in time they came from a culture that was different from what we now know as mainstream American.

The health education curricula of the '90s and beyond must be all inclusive, not exclusive. That is, it should be inclusive in the sense that all human beings have a need to deal with health issues, regardless of their backgrounds, values, and beliefs. Self-esteem is a major component of wellness. Without positive self-esteem, persons suffer a variety of illnesses that range from mental/emotional to physical problems. An inclusive program is one that teaches students to accept and appreciate themselves with all their strengths and weaknesses. It is one in which students learn to see other people as having equal worth and dignity regardless of their backgrounds. In essence, cultural and linguistic inclusion allows for all students to equally benefit from their experiences in school and the community at large.

Another key element in a comprehensive health education program is for the teachers to have high expectations for all students, regardless of background or ability. There is no room for prejudice or stereotypes. The teacher should serve as mediator of the learning process, providing the best opportunities for each student to realize his/her potential in the classroom. A comprehensive health education program can allow for a wide array of stimulating activities that provide the backdrop for teaching all content areas in a positive way.

It is important to prepare relevant, motivating materials and activities for students. Based on the students' concerns and interests that the teacher has identified, materials can be adapted to make instruction more meaningful and exciting. When possible, students should also assist in the creation of their own materials.

Liberal use of a variety of instructional materials helps all students learn more effectively, but is particularly helpful for those youngsters for whom English is not their primary language. Materials should reflect cultural and gender equity, grade-level and linguistic appropriateness, and interesting content. When developing or reviewing materials, keep the following criteria in mind:

- Materials contain no labels or stereotypes demeaning of any cultural or ethnic group.
- Materials display all groups in a variety of professions or occupations.
- Materials present contributions and achievements of all groups.
- Materials depict differences in customs and beliefs as desirable.
- Materials contain equal representation of all groups in mental and physical activities.
- Materials show socioeconomic ranges for all groups.
- Materials reflect a balance of both traditional and nontraditional family compositions.

Conclusion

If comprehensive health education is truly going to reflect the reality of the multicultural society that has always existed in America, a considerable amount of effort must be made to develop and/or adapt health education curricula, as it exists today. A reexamination of values and beliefs should take place, and a sincere attempt at celebrating diversity must occur in schools and communities across the nation. The tapestry of cultures and languages that exist in this country can be a positive driving force in developing healthy and productive lifestyles among all people. Through health education, students and families can learn to eliminate racism and prejudice, violence and crime, illness and disease, poverty and misery. The schools and communities in America must stop the denial of this country's diversity and not force people to give up their differences in exchange for access to the society. Health and wellness affects everyone, and schools have a responsibility to deal with health education in a comprehensive manner.

References

Council on Scientific Affairs. 1991. Hispanic health in the United States. *JAMA* 265 (2): 248-252.

De La Rosa, D., and C. Maw. 1990. *Hispanic education: A statistical portrait.* Washington, DC: National Council of La Raza.

De La Torre, A. 1993. Access is vital in health-care reform. *Los Angeles Times,* 31 March.

English, J., A. Sancho, D. Lloyd-Kolkin and L. Hunter. 1990. *Criteria for comprehensive health education curricula.* Los Alamitos, CA: Southwest Regional Laboratory.

Johnson, J., and A. Kernan-Schloss. 1992. *Faulty diagnosis: Public misconceptions about health care reform.* New York: The Public Agenda Foundation.

Maxwell, B., and M. Jacobson. 1989. *Marketing disease to Hispanics.* Washington, DC: Center for Science in the Public Interest.

National Council of La Raza. 1991. Hispanic child poverty: Signs of distress, signs of hope. *NCLR Agenda* 10 (2): 15-17.

Rubin, R., D. Moran, K. Jones and M. Hackbarth. 1988. *Critical conditions: America's health care in jeopardy.* Washington, DC: National Committee for Quality Health Care.

Sancho, A., J. English, L. Hunter and D. Lloyd-Kolkin. 1991. *Comprehensive school health education for Hispanic youth: Insights about curriculum adaptation.* Los Alamitos, CA: Southwest Regional Laboratory.

Sancho, A., B. De La Rocha, L. Hunter and D. Lloyd-Kolkin. 1992. *Hispanic health education activities for youth and their parents.* Los Alamitos, CA: Southwest Regional Laboratory.

Stolberg, S. 1992. Fatalismo toward cancer. *Los Angeles Times*, 26 December.

Chapter 6

General Guidelines for an Effective and Culturally Sensitive Approach to Health Education

Sally M. Davis, PhD, CHES

Designing and implementing effective health education that is culturally sensitive can be challenging to even the most experienced and well-meaning health educator. The success of a program depends on building a strong foundation that includes a clearly articulated rationale, a theoretical framework, and a combination of approaches gleaned from other successful programs and developed in partnership with local communities. This chapter discusses these essential components and gives an example of a health education curriculum that integrates them into a successful program.

Rationale for Designing Culturally Sensitive Health Education

The leading causes of morbidity and mortality in the United States have changed over the past thirty years. There has been a significant decrease in the rate of mortality from infectious diseases. Conversely, the rate of mortality related to behavioral, social, or lifestyle factors has increased. The dramatic lowering of mortality rates is evident for all populations in the United States, although the rate for minorities remains significantly higher than that of nonminorities (Public Health Service, Health Resources and Service Administration, 1991).

Therapeutic medicine and improved sanitation have been relatively successful in reducing infectious disease. The most dramatic example is the effective treatment of tuberculosis among Navajo Indians in the southwestern United States where there was a marked decrease in mortality between 1950 and 1959 even without any significant improvement in economic situation. Yet even as deaths from infectious disease declined, noninfectious illness and mortality increased in absolute and relative significance. This rise in lifestyle diseases has caused many to question the efficacy of medicine alone in preventing or curing those diseases that result from social and personal conditions, termed the "new morbidity" (Haggerty, 1977).

The recognition that medicine alone is not enough has led to a nationwide public health initiative. In July 1979, the publication *Healthy People: The Surgeon General's Report on Health Promotion and Disease Prevention* described for the first time a national public health agenda. This report established five quantifiable goals for improving the health of all Americans and documented the importance of disease prevention and health promotion in achieving these goals (Haggerty, 1977). In 1980, *Promoting Health/Preventing Disease: Objectives for the Nation* was published as a companion document. This plan of action listed 226 measurable objectives that called for improvements in health status, risk reduction, public and professional awareness, health services and protective measures, and surveillance and evaluation (Public Health Service, 1979).

Although progress in achieving those earlier objectives was documented in areas such as hypertension, childhood infectious diseases and injury prevention (Public Health Service, 1980; Centers for Disease Control and Prevention, 1987, 1988a, 1988b), new public health challenges became apparent. Therefore, in 1987, the Public Health Service (PHS) began developing the objectives for the year 2000. The U.S. Secretary of Health and Human Services and the National Academy of Sciences' Institute of Medicine organized a consortium of more than 300 national organizations and state and territorial health departments to work on the project. The resulting publication, *Healthy People 2000: National Health Promotion and Disease Prevention Objectives* (U.S. Department of health and Human Services, 1991), launched "a national strategy for significantly improving the health of the Nation over the coming decade."

Three basic goals of *Healthy People 2000* are to increase the span of healthy life for Americans; to reduce health disparities among Americans; and to achieve access to preventive services for all Americans. Measurable objectives to be achieved by the year 2000 are organized into four categories:

- health promotion strategies that relate to individual lifestyle
- health protection strategies that relate to environmental or regulatory measures
- preventive services that include counseling, screening, immunization or chemoprophylactic intervention
- morbidity and mortality surveillance and data systems

The American Association of School Administrators is one of nine national groups chosen by the U.S. Public Health Service to help promote *Healthy People 2000*. In the foreword to that group's *Action Plan for Schools* (American Association of School Administrators, 1991), Executive Director Richard D. Miller calls for leaders of the nation's schools to make children's health a priority. He states:

> Schools reach 95 percent of children. We, as school leaders, have the greatest opportunity to teach children about personal responsibility for health. They must know with no uncertainty how their daily decisions about diet, smoking, exercise, alcohol and drug use, sexual activity, and safety will have an impact on the extent to which they will live happy, productive, and fulfilling lives. Their future and our futures depend on it.

In many communities in the United States today, schools have a major role in providing public health education to the members of the community as well as to children in the classroom. Children from the ages of five through eighteen spend the majority of their time each day in school. Therefore, contact with all children for an extended period of time is possible. In addition, the school is an important centralized facility available for after school health education activities for the entire family. School administration and other relevant staff can serve as facilitators and role models.

Theoretical Base for Designing Culturally Sensitive Health Education

A wide range of social scientists, physicians and educators have suggested many causes for the high rate of preventable diseases, injuries and death among minority populations. Despair and low self-esteem resulting from a lack of social and economic opportunity and persistent poverty are frequently cited. Some authors indicate that local customs may operate against certain types of achievement and success. In some communities offering to help someone with a personal issue may be viewed as meddling or interference. Other professionals believe that social disintegration and acculturation pressures associated with economic development are to blame. Not to be overlooked is the fact that many minority people have survived a history of oppression—they have been rejected and marginalized from society for generations (Drinnon, 1980). Certainly this exclusion of minorities must contribute to a collective as well as individual sense of powerlessness and lack of self-efficacy on their part.

A key ingredient in changing health behaviors is self-efficacy—the confidence a person feels about performing a particular activity. Not only is it important for people to want to change their behavior, but they must feel they can. Albert Bandura explains in his social cognitive theory that the inability to influence events and social conditions that significantly affect one's life can give rise to feelings of futility and despondency, as well as to anxiety (Bandura, 1986). People may give up trying because they seriously doubt they can do what is required. Or they may be assured of their capabilities but give up trying because they expect that their efforts will not produce any results due to an unresponsive, negatively biased, or punitive social environment. These two separate sources of futility have quite different causes and remedial implications. Bandura analyzes self-efficacy as a developmental process starting with children in their family, peer and school contexts and continuing during childhood, adolescence, adulthood, and old age.

Bandura further states that personal efficacy leads to collective efficacy and social change. People do not live their lives in social isolation. Many of the challenges and difficulties they face reflect group problems requiring sustained collective effort to produce significant change. The strength of groups, organizations, and even nations lies partly in people's sense of collective efficacy. They believe that they can solve their problems and improve their lives through concerted effort. They must feel empowered to break the cycle of stress- and grief-producing situations that are the products as well as the causative agents in this reciprocative environment. Empowerment as used here is defined as a social action process that promotes participation of people, organizations and communities in gaining control over their lives in their community and larger society (Wallerstein and Bernstein, 1988). With this perspective, empowerment is not characterized as achieving power to dominate others, but rather power to act with others to effect change. Any community action process such as comprehensive health education must be done within a cultural context.

Culture refers to the patterns of behavior and belief common to members of a society. It is the basis for establishing rules for understanding and generating customary behavior. Culture includes beliefs, norms, values, assumptions, expectations and plans for action. It is the framework within which people see the world around them, interpret events and behavior, and react to their perceived reality. It is important that the health educator understand these basic concepts of culture and consider the following steps in designing culturally sensitive health education programs:

1. Identify community contacts and resources, develop linkages, and build proactive partnerships to include the multiple populations, sectors and systems within a community to address health education needs and concerns.
2. Establish a community advisory group or steering committee to guide the direction of the program planners.
3. Conduct a needs assessment to identify concerns and determine priorities in order to characterize the need and plan appropriate services.

4. Conduct surveys to collect information on sociodemographic characteristics and family histories.
5. Conduct focus groups to determine perceived needs, "generative themes" (topics people feel strongly about), formal and informal structures, community assets, identity of change agents and other information crucial to program and evaluation design.
6. Implement a pilot project.
7. Document all activities for the purpose of evaluation.

Focus Groups—The Link to Community Opinions

Perhaps the most important step a health educator can take when designing a culturally sensitive program is to implement focus groups. Focus groups are an important tool in designing, implementing and evaluating the curriculum and have been used extensively with teachers, parents, students and other community members. A focus group, group interview or group discussion focuses on a particular topic—usually a response to a situation or issue such as smoking or drug use. The group is also focused in the sense that instead of a group of mixed people, each group is made up of people with things in common. This common focus can be people from the same age group, the same gender, or the same role (Hawe, Degeling and Hall, 1990).

Focus groups are a relatively simple way to collect more information from the target group. Using a discussion outline or issue menu, information is elicited from the group on a given topic or situation. The group facilitator keeps the session on track, while still allowing people to talk freely and spontaneously. This draws out the range of perceptions and beliefs in the group. This information can guide the health educator in making decisions that reflect the cultural milieu of the community. The focus group is one of the methods used when a range of opinion is the principal goal.

A focus group enables the health educator to gain a broad understanding of why participants think and act the way they do (Hawe, Degeling and Hall, 1990). Conducting focus groups will assist in understanding the range of different attitudes toward a topic and help the health educator explore the reasons behind people's attitudes and behavior. Qualitative data collected from a focus group can provide a basis to develop a questionnaire for a quantitative survey (Krueger, 1988). This approach is particularly useful in the planning stages of program development in health education.

Since focus groups are not always the most appropriate method for collecting community opinion and can be time consuming and expensive, the health educator needs to answer the following questions before initiating focus groups:

1. Is it worthwhile to use focus groups or group interviews in this situation?
2. Who would be a part of the group or groups?
3. How many groups would be conducted?
4. How will participants be recruited?
5. What incentives could be used?
6. Where is an acceptable and convenient place to conduct the focus groups?

The Interview Protocol
An interview protocol is an outline of the questions and issues to be discussed in the focus group. Each question should cover a specific issue and be broad enough to evoke a group response. The health educator should be prepared with background information about the target group and the concerns that affect them in order

to anticipate some of the issues. The protocol should include open-ended questions and may include prompts and other information to help the group facilitator achieve smooth discussion and draw people out.

The first question is particularly important and should be one that is likely to include all members of the group. Questions should be arranged so that each subsequent question narrows the issues, and the discussion flows from a question to an answer that pertains to the next question. If each new question changes the topic and breaks the flow it creates confusion. It is also important that the most sensitive questions are discussed last. This happens anyway if the questions are funneled from the beginning. It is helpful to have a representative from the culture of the target community to help write the questions.

The Focus Group Facilitator

The role of the focus group facilitator is to elicit information from group members, while at the same time preventing sidetracking or domination of the group's discussion by any one member. It is important that the facilitator be familiar with the subject area in order to differentiate between important and unimportant avenues of discussion. However, the facilitator need not be an expert in the field.

During the focus group session, the facilitator should not express strong opinions about the topic area in order to avoid influencing or curbing the information provided by the group. The facilitator should treat all participants equally, avoid belittling anyone and avoid giving answers. The facilitator should remain neutral and not agree or disagree with anyone's comments. At the same time, the facilitator will need to maintain discipline, and prevent dominance of the group by any member(s) who may want to hold center stage.

The facilitator should establish an atmosphere of trust and mutual respect that puts people at ease, and provides the basis for free-flowing, spontaneous discussion. He or she should emphasize that there are no right or wrong answers and should encourage the expression of different opinions and perceptions.

Preparation for the Focus Group

Before the participants arrive, the facilitator should prepare name tags and make seating arrangements. Name tags or table tents (place cards) will help the facilitator to address individuals directly. Seating is very important since some seats may allow for ready eye-contact with the moderator while others may not. The seats should be arranged before the session so that each participant will have the same line of view.

Leading the Focus Group

Group participants should be seated in a circle or semicircle or around a table. Facilitators should set the stage by introducing themselves and explaining their role and nonexpert status. They should, however, display a certain degree of authority on procedural matters. Time should be taken to explain the purpose of the group, the agenda for the discussion, and the rules for the session. Rules that should be mentioned include the expectation that all members of the group will have a say, people should not speak at the same time, people should say what they think and not what they think someone else wants to hear, and that there are no right or wrong answers. The facilitator should reiterate that he or she is interested in the range of opinions and differing points of view. This is a good time to mention that the session will be recorded on tape and that detailed notes will be taken. Remind participants that responses will be treated with confidentiality and that no information will be identified by individual source.

To begin the group, have everyone introduce themselves and offer some information about themselves that relates to the purpose of the group. The facilitator should then proceed to the interview protocol using the first question as a "warm-up." Following the predetermined list of questions will help keep the group focused, but the facilitator must permit and elicit a wide range of responses. The facilitator must listen perceptively so that exploration of new areas can be possible, while at the same time probe to encourage specificity. Distractions should be discouraged while encouraging the involvement of all participants.

Closing the Focus Group

If there is time, the facilitator may want to summarize the main points and suggestions discussed, and list them on a flip chart or blackboard. This will leave the participants with the feeling that their contributions will be valued and taken seriously. However, in cases where there is not consensus on critical issues—or for other reasons—it may be preferable not to draw conclusions. Each individual focus group should be made aware that it has a limited contribution to the decision-making process, and participants should not get the impression that the issues have been decided by them. After the group is formally concluded, the facilitator should thank the members for their participation and contribution and tell them someone will be contacting them regarding future focus group meetings.

An Example of a Culturally Sensitive Health Education Curriculum

This example of a culturally sensitive health education program was designed to reduce risk factors for chronic disease by developing lifelong health habits through a school-based curriculum. Few curriculum models are available for special populations. Curricula designed for homogeneous classrooms are unintentionally ethnocentric and inappropriate for many of the students in the multicultural classroom. Local beliefs and customs may be overlooked or ignored. The project may be viewed with suspicion if it has been devised and established without these considerations.

The following example is based on the premise that empowerment leads to self-efficacy and in turn produces healthful behavioral changes. Understanding the cultural context of the community has been key in designing this curriculum. Intergenerational activities strengthen self-concept and cultural identity. Multidisciplinary planning through group process has provided a synergistic and comprehensive approach. Including traditions/customs throughout the curriculum builds self-esteem and provides a sense of continuity. Intercultural communication techniques have been used to provide skills necessary for understanding and tolerance. Emphasis has been placed on identifying and supporting cultural role models who have healthy lifestyles.

Pathways to Health is a program funded by the National Institutes of Health, National Cancer Institute (#CA52283) and developed at the Center for Indian Youth Program Development under the leadership of Sally Davis and Leslie Cunningham-Sabo. Unlike most health education programs at the elementary and middle school level, *Pathways to Health* was developed especially for and with input from the target population. American Indian health educators, researchers, teachers and advisors contributed to the overall design and content. Traditional customs and values were woven into the fabric of the program. For example, traditional foods such as corn, beans and squash that are low in fat and high in fiber are emphasized along with other foods first cultivated by Native Americans. The rich heritage of stories, poems, songs and games regarding healthful living and foodways were used as a resource.

Elders from the local communities have been included as teachers in the curriculum to teach the children about traditional Native American ways that recognize the importance of taking measures to prevent illness and promote a healthful lifestyle. For example, one Pueblo grandfather pointing out the window says, "You see all these fields, they used to be used to grow food for people. Now all these fields are used to grow food for cows." This illustrates a very poignant example of the agricultural change from growing produce to raising beef and a dietary change from one high in vegetables and grains to one high in beef. Students learn that game such as buffalo and venison is leaner than beef and that a four-ounce serving of buffalo steak contains only about two grams of fat, compared to ten grams in a similar serving of beef sirloin steak (choice grade). Lessons explain that wild animals do not usually get fat, and their meat is only slightly marbled. Also discussed is the great expenditure of energy required for hunting and that every hunt did not always result in meat on the table, so meat was not usually consumed daily. These discussions do not imply that it would be best to return to the old ways, but rather integrate historically valuable information into the lessons in ways that validate the culture of the students.

The concepts taught in the *Pathways to Health* curriculum are reinforced through activities in science, social studies, mathematics and language arts. Music and art activities are also included. This integrated approach makes the curriculum very attractive to classroom teachers who usually feel more comfortable teaching these core subjects than they do teaching health. By specifically addressing the New Mexico Department of Education Competencies in the curriculum, the effort to teach the required course of study is given priority.

Teachers are trained during a two-day session held at the University of New Mexico. They may register for university credit, and if they complete the full two days of training and teach the curriculum they receive one unit credit in health education. The educators' training includes the rationale, content and teaching methods of the curriculum. Sample lessons are modeled and elders from representative communities give an example of an inter-generational lesson. An intercultural communication workshop is included so teachers have an opportunity to practice new communication skills and explore different cultural issues.

School staff members (classroom teachers, school nurses and school food service personnel) have been incorporated into the *Pathways to Health* program in order to enhance acceptance of the program in the schools and promote continuance of the program after the project staff departs. Support activities include staff development, coaching, model teaching and provision of materials. Effective instructional materials were developed based on an understanding of teachers' needs and the use of focus groups. The process of implementing and institutionalizing the program into the schools is being evaluated using the concerns-based approach developed by Hall and Hord (1987).

Group process was used extensively in the development of the curriculum and evaluation instruments. A multicultural, multi-disciplinary research team from the Center for Indian Youth Program Development in the Department of Pediatrics at the University of New Mexico School of Medicine worked together to ensure that the lessons were developmentally, educationally, culturally and scientifically accurate and germane. The result has been a highly successful curriculum well accepted by the students and their teachers and parents.

Conclusion

When faced with the challenge of designing and implementing a comprehensive health education program that is culturally sensitive, it is important to clearly articulate the rationale for the program in terms of the perceived as well as the documented needs of the community. From this point a strong theoretical framework and a variety of workable approaches from which to proceed must be developed. The most essential ingredient in a successful program for special populations is a viable partnership with the community. This chapter has discussed some of the methods for developing a community partnership. Focus groups have been shown to be a valuable link to community opinions and guidance.

Pathways to Health is a health promotion curriculum for American Indian students. This curriculum was developed in partnership with Native American communities using the approaches discussed in this chapter.

References

American Association of School Administrators. 1991. *Healthy kids for the year 2000: An action plan for schools*. Arlington, VA.

Bandura, A. 1986. *Social foundations of thoughts and actions: A social cognitive theory*. New York: Prentice Hall.

Centers for Disease Control and Prevention. 1987. Advancements in meeting the 1990 hypertension objectives. *Morbidity and Mortality Weekly Report* 36:144, 149-151.

Centers for Disease Control and Prevention. 1988a. Progress toward achieving the national 1990 objectives for immunization. *Morbidity and Mortality Weekly Report* 37:613-617.

Centers for Disease Control and Prevention. 1988b. Progress toward achieving the national 1990 objectives for injury prevention and control. *Morbidity and Mortality Weekly Report* 37:138-140, 145-149.

Drinnon, R. 1980. *Facing West: The metaphysics of Indian-hating and empire-building*. New York: Meridian Books.

Haggerty, R. J. 1977. Changing lifestyles to improve health. *Preventive Medicine* 6:276-289.

Hall, G., and S. Hord. 1987. *Change in schools: Facilitating the process.* Albany, NY: State University of New York Press.

Hawe, P., D. Degeling and J. Hall. 1990. *Evaluating health promotion: A health worker's guide.* Sidney, Australia: Maclennan and Petty.

Krueger, R. 1988. *Focus groups: A practical guide for applied research.* Newbury Park, CA: Sage Publications.

Public Health Service. 1979. *Healthy people: The surgeon general's report on health promotion and disease prevention.* DHEW Publication No. (PHS)79-55071. Washington, DC: U. S. Department of Health, Education and Welfare.

Public Health Service. 1980. *Promoting health/preventing disease: Objectives for the nation.* Washington, DC: U.S. Department of Health and Human Services.

Public Health Service, Health Resources and Services Administration. 1991. *Health status of minorities and low-income groups: Third Edition.* Washington, DC: U.S. Department of Health and Human Services.

U.S. Department of Health and Human Services, Public Health Service. 1991. *Healthy people 2000: National health promotion and disease prevention objectives.* DHHS Publication No. (PHS) 91-50212. Washington, DC.

Wallerstein, N., and E. Bernstein. 1988. Breaking new ground for youth at risk: Prevention theory and research related to high-risk youth. *Office of Substance Abuse Technical Report* 1:380.

Chapter 7

Integrating Multicultural Health Education into the Curriculum

Markella L. Pahnos, PhD,
and Karen L. Butt, EdD

The United States is composed of many different cultural and ethnic groups. Most of these groups are given inequitable attention in school environments including the make-up of faculty, texts, other teaching related materials and curricula. Most curricula focus on the dominant cultural group, frequently referred to as mainstream America. When the curriculum focuses predominantly on the experiences of one group, all students, including those from the mainstream, suffer negative consequences.

A mainstream-centric curriculum denies students the chance to experience and grow from knowledge, perspectives and frames of reference from cultures and groups other than their own. This can contribute to a misleading concept of one's own culture and its relationship with other cultural, racial and ethnic groups. Additionally, a mainstream-centric curriculum denies students the opportunity to view their culture from the perspectives of other groups. When given this opportunity to view their own culture from another's point of view, they may be better able to understand their own culture more fully. They may discover its uniqueness, see how it differs from others, and learn to understand how it relates to and interacts with them (Banks, 1991).

Curriculum Defined

A curriculum, in its broadest sense, influences and is influenced by the entire school environment. Curricula, therefore, must be viewed as all the experiences, both planned and unplanned that learners are exposed to under the umbrella of the school. Following this definition, a multicultural curriculum, in its broadest sense, embraces all diversity from cultural differences to sexual preferences.

What Makes a Health Curriculum Multicultural?

While health education is only one subject area, its curriculum must also address broader issues such as teachers' values and expectations, student cliques and peer groupings, school regulations, individual learning styles, and the perceptions that all students and teachers bring to the school. Therefore, cultural pluralism should permeate the entire curriculum. According to Banks (1981), to accomplish this the health education curriculum must

- promote values, attitudes and behaviors that support cultural pluralism
- reflect the cultural learning styles of all students
- provide students with continuous opportunities to develop a better sense of self
- help students understand the totality of experiences related to their health and well-being
- teach conflict resolution skills
- develop decision-making skills, social-participation skills and a sense of political efficacy

- foster positive multicultural interactions between health teachers and students
- develop skills necessary for both interpersonal and intercultural interaction
- make maximum use of local and community resources
- use assessment procedures that reflect students' cultural preferences
- have ongoing formative evaluation of the curriculum

The Curriculum Committee

The school is the traditional arena where teaching and learning take place. The school has numerous responsibilities to children and their parents in regard to all health issues. The administrator's responsibility is to ensure a healthy school environment, to provide needed health services and high quality and appropriate health instruction. The first step to providing quality health instruction is to develop a sound and applicable health curriculum.

The work of planning, writing and revising curriculum should be a responsibility shared by the home, the school and the community (Redican, Olsen and Baffi, 1993). The home is important because it is the primary source for the development of children's values and beliefs. These values differ from culture to culture and must be considered in curriculum planning. Schools should develop an open-door policy with parents and encourage their participation in school activities. School officials should do all they can to solicit parent involvement and support. This is most important in culturally diverse areas (Redican, Olsen and Baffi, 1993).

All children are part of the community in which they live. The community can support the curriculum in numerous ways. They can contribute monies, resources and support for health issues and projects. Additionally, the community can contribute real learning experiences enabling students to practice healthy living skills.

To begin this process schools should have a curriculum development committee consisting of the principal, health education coordinator, health instructors, school nurse, guidance counselor, parents and appropriate community members. It would be beneficial to have representation from the various diverse groups on this committee. Additionally, there must be an orientation to prepare all those involved in the planning to think and act multiculturally.

The principal is generally the primary administrator on the curriculum committee and it is his or her responsibility to promote optimal learning for all students. In some school districts, the health education coordinator is also an administrator. The coordinator is responsible for health instruction for the district and coordination of educational efforts.

The health instructors use their strategies and knowledge to ensure that the curriculum is taught and that this instruction is culturally diverse. The guidance counselor considers the emotional climate in which the instruction takes place. The parents provide understanding and support for individual differences and needs expressed by the home. Finally, the community lends support for the differences and similarities that influence health instruction.

The promotion, protection and maintenance of the health and well-being of children require the coordinated efforts of the school, community groups and individuals. If this coordination does not occur, curricula will remain mainstream-centric.

Identifying Community Health Needs

Why should we involve the community in health education? School health education programs cannot be developed in isolation without regard for the community and expect to be meaningful and applicable in assessing the community's health and cultural needs. The following questions should be considered (Pollock, 1987):

- Who are the people living in the community?
- How many are parents of school-age children?
- How many single-parent homes are there?
- What is the population of racial/ethnic students?
- To what ethnic and cultural groups do the heads of households belong?
- What is the preferred method of communication within the various community groups?
- What are the expectations and attitudes of the people?

Identifying Individual and Special Health Needs

Because the curriculum is being planned for a specific population it is important that their health and cultural needs be examined and addressed. These needs can be determined through direct observation as well as information gathered from various groups and student health records. While addressing the specific cultural needs of the area it is important not to become ethnocentric and overlook or exclude national and global health issues from the curriculum.

Planning to Meet Legal Requirements

The planning committee must consider any and all state or school mandates and requirements that must be included in the curriculum. Currently, few mandates for inclusion of diversity issues in school curricula exist. Most multicultural requirements tend to be found in major city school districts rather than in state mandates.

Curriculum Revision

Unfortunately, history shows us that multicultural curriculum revision has frequently been a mere superficial addendum to the predominantly mainstream-centric curriculum. Too often, a Black-American history week or a Chinese New Year celebration has been tagged on to the existing curriculum rather than carrying out complete curriculum revision which should include changing fundamental objectives and adding perspectives from minority groups.

Several reasons for this shortcoming have been suggested, including the assumption among many educators and administrators that a multicultural curriculum is only legitimate or necessary for those minorities represented in given communities. This explains how the monocultural ideologies continue to dominate and permeate American curricula. Schools must practice multicultural education regardless of whether the student and faculty populations are homogeneous or heterogeneous. The success or failure of educators to do this greatly influences the shaping of student learning and behavior. Additionally, many curriculum committees lack the exposure, background and necessary skills to enable them to incorporate multiculturalism into their curricula (Gay, 1988).

Considering Available Curricula
There are numerous excellent curricula available for health education and some interesting general multicultural curricula. It is not always necessary to write a curriculum from the beginning. It is possible, and often times preferable, to revise and rewrite an existing curriculum. The most important factor is that the curriculum is the correct match between the students' backgrounds and needs.

Curriculum Planning and Development

Multicultural curriculum planning must go across the curriculum on each level. A strong multicultural base or foundation must be established in the early years so that as students move through the curriculum and grade levels it can be built upon. Additionally, a true picture of multiculturalism cannot be taught in a specific topic or content area alone. It should permeate the entire curriculum and cross disciplines (i.e., topics, content and subject areas).

The existing health education curriculum should be appraised before revision, writing or rewriting takes place. This appraisal should determine whether or not the curriculum meets the students' current and future health needs, whether it addresses cultural diversity and how the two can be blended together.

Integrated Versus Separate Subject

Two different philosophies exist in terms of multicultural curricula. One is that ethnic pluralism should permeate not only the entire curriculum, but rather the total school environment. Banks and Banks (1993) describe four levels of integration of multicultural content:

- Level one, the *contribution's approach*, is the most basic and focuses on simple areas such as heroes and holidays.
- Level two, the *additive approach*, looks at adding to the curriculum without changing its structure.
- Level three, the *transformation approach*, changes the structure to enable students to view several aspects of diverse cultural groups.
- Level four, the *social action approach*, enables students to make decisions and problem-solve about multicultural issues.

Deciding the level of multicultural integration is a vital first step when writing or revising health curricula. It is important to note that when a curriculum is integrated throughout, it is hard to evaluate what and how much is being assimilated. Therefore, some schools opt to take the easier route of creating a separate portion of the curriculum devoted only to multicultural issues.

While this is obviously easier to evaluate, it perpetuates the concept that multiculturalism is a separate issue and not a whole part of society and health.

Rationale and/or Philosophy

Given the broad nature of most health curricula, multiculturalism can easily be incorporated into an existing philosophy. However, before a philosophy can be developed or curriculum design reformed, schools must evaluate current monocultural and ethnocentric biases and practices. Once this issue is addressed, the school community can then begin to refine the underlying philosophy that will guide curriculum reform.

Without a guiding philosophy, teaching and learning become aimless, haphazard and possibly useless. Multiculturalism must be the force that directs all philosophy and curricular decisions in order to offer equity in education to all students.

Scope and Sequence

All curricula should be planned sequentially. Just as with K through 12 comprehensive health lessons, the multicultural components must also build one concept upon another. The concepts and behavior should reflect the maturity and readiness of the student throughout. Multicultural education as a part of health education should strive to prevent the formation of negative habits, attitudes and behaviors rather than try to change them once they are already established. Therefore, this education must begin in preschool and be carried on throughout the entire school experience.

Goals and Objectives

Because goals are long-range and general in focus, it is important that multicultural components be included in these broad statements. Additionally, multiculturalism should be included in all three of the domains: cognitive, affective and active. It is tempting to think that multicultural lessons should fall within the affective domain only; but this is not the case, and the temptation to write only affective goals should be avoided.

The objectives should present clear and precise means by which to reach the goals. They must address through action steps ways to achieve multicultural health education. They should include such issues as the following:

- generating ethnic-specific content and experiences
- creating experiences that help students with their own identity and feelings toward other groups
- clarifying unjust feelings towards others
- attaining a balanced perspective of one's own cultural group
- addressing other cultural groups; developing a global sense
- attaining a balance of cross-cultural skills

Content

Health education is a dynamic rather than static subject in which the curricula content considers all dimensions of the physical, mental, social, emotional and spiritual being. This person, however, is also unique because of his or her race, sex, culture and special needs.

Choosing content when culture focuses on a body of traditions, customs and practices, and the history or the knowledge of a people, can result in a curriculum which focuses heavily on the cultural content of one or more specific groups, causing it to be static. However, if culture is seen as a continuing creation of different peoples, building on the past and moving toward the future, then the curriculum is process-oriented and dynamic, enabling health educators to integrate the two.

Critical issues such as hunger, teen pregnancy, suicide, substance use, child abuse and violence must be considered simultaneously with multiculturalism and diversity. Multicultural health education must focus more closely on the individual and examine issues such as self-esteem, family structures, male and female roles, and the belief and value structures of students and how these affect behavior and wellness (Pahnos, 1992).

Figure 1, the Multicultural Health Education Model, depicts how the health content areas fit together like pieces of a puzzle within the wellness triangle. Surrounding the triangle are the diverse influences of the individual, peers, family, school and community, beyond the community and global. This model illustrates how all of these influences can form a cohesive bond to collectively incorporate the various health areas and aspects of each child's world and beyond. This visualization should enable the curriculum planner and writer to more clearly understand how multicultural issues must permeate the entire curriculum.

Organizing Learning Experiences

When organizing learning experiences and choosing instructional strategies, it is easy to get stuck at the level of games, foods and customs. Prejudice reduction should be the predominant goal of multicultural education rather than aiming for these soft targets (Pahnos and Butt, 1992). Methods and activities must build upon each other and be ongoing rather than mere appendages. Lessons must fit the teacher's style of teaching and philosophy. It is the teacher's task to come to grips with his or her biases and prejudices, to take a stand and to decide whether to be a part of the problem or a part of the solution (Bateman, 1974).

Health education that is multicultural must include skills such as decision making and problem solving as vehicles to change. Banks and Banks (1993) state that these skills provide for the greatest level of integration of multicultural content.

Identifying Resources and Materials

Schools and the curriculum planning committee should at the very least set up guidelines for teachers to analyze appropriate bias-free materials. These guidelines should be used for any resources and/or materials listed in the curriculum. Major criteria for evaluating health education resources listed by Ames, Trucano, Wan and Harris (1992) include freedom from cultural, ethnic,

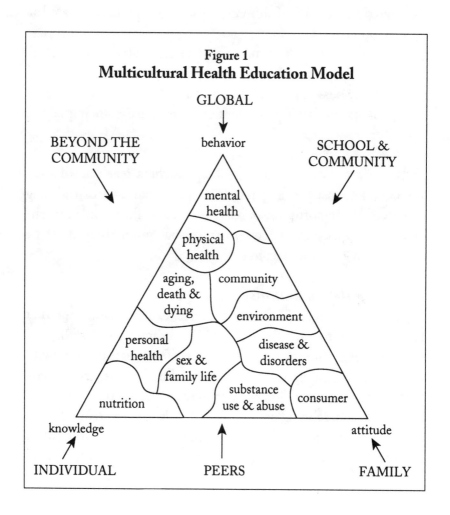

Figure 1
Multicultural Health Education Model

age, racial, disability, sexual orientation and sex bias. They also list the following questions for evaluating resources for bias:

• Does the material include a variety of groups?
• Does it include multiethnic content appropriate to the population?

Are both males and females depicted as worthy role models?
• Is there a balance between male and female content?
• Are contributions of different ethnic groups incorporated in the content?
• Are the resources and materials free from stereotyping of all kinds?
• Are older persons depicted positively?
• Are individuals with disabilities shown using their positive skills?

Resources should be used to help teachers reach all of their students, not just the majority for a particular area or the long accepted White norm. Resources can make a difference in teaching, and if they are to have instructional merit, they must be culturally diverse and bias free.

Involving the Community

Schools do not have all of the resources, expertise and time that children need to provide them with lifetime health skills and behaviors. For this reason schools must form partnerships with community members to ensure that children will receive maximum health benefits. These collaborations must take place between children, schools, community organizations and businesses. If schools are to reduce bias this collaboration must occur between all of the different races, cultures, sexes, ages and mentally and physically challenged individuals in the community.

Identifying Problem Areas

Parents and communities have different views regarding the role of the school in their children's education. There are those individuals who believe that education should remain a "melting pot" and that students should adopt the health beliefs and behaviors of the dominant culture. While others claim that schools and curricula should be using the "tossed salad approach" where individual differences are appreciated as an integral part of the whole (Airhihenbuwa and Pineiro, 1988). Controversies arise when these views come into opposition with one another. Ames et al. (1992) provide three steps for preventing controversies:

- Adhere to an open and systematic curriculum-planning process.
- Assign qualified teachers to teach health and train them to handle sensitive issues.
- Develop policies and procedures for dealing with controversial issues.

Curriculum Implementation

This is perhaps the most difficult part of the curriculum process. This is the part where the plans must now be put into action. If the curriculum planning committee did their work thoroughly and all of the preceding steps were followed, the plan should work. However, if vital sections were overlooked and missing, the plan may never become reality. It is all too easy for administration to retreat to the traditional curriculum which may have gone unchallenged for years. At this point multicultural curricula are for the most part new frontiers in education and sure to be challenged. Therefore, it is prudent for the curriculum to cover all areas to make implementation as smooth and easy as possible.

Curriculum Evaluation

Evaluation must be used to determine both strengths and weaknesses of the educational process. Once these two facets have been identified, then revision and reinforcement can occur (Redican, Olsen and Baffi, 1993). To evaluate whether the health curriculum responds to and reflects the ethnic and cultural diversity of students and society, the following set of questions may be helpful:

- Do the books and other materials to be used reflect diversity (e.g., ethnicity, sex, age, various physical disabilities, class)? Are different groups portrayed honestly, realistically and sensitively?
- Do the curriculum writers know the children for whom the curriculum is being written? How will it use their backgrounds, values and ways of thinking to improve instruction?
- When developing goals and strategies, did the curriculum committee consider the different cultures and learning styles of the children?
- Will the curriculum help the children learn to function effectively in different cultures?
- Will the curriculum help strengthen children's sense of identity? Will it help them understand themselves better in light of their own heritage?
- Will the curriculum include discussions about prejudice and discrimination?
- Will the curriculum include positive and negative aspects of ethnic group experiences? (Matiella, 1991)

Additionally, the following questions can be used to facilitate the evaluation process of curriculum components:
- Does the curriculum rationale reflect sensitivity to and celebration of various kinds of diversifying factors among students?

- Does diversity permeate the core of the appropriate curriculum components, especially the content and activities?
- Does the pluralistic content included play a central role and function in understanding [health] subject matter?
- Is the pluralistic content used as the context or arena for major skill development?
- Will students from different ethnic and cultural backgrounds find the proposed instructional materials personally meaningful to their life experiences?
- Has a wide variety of culturally different examples, situations, scenarios and anecdotes been used throughout the curriculum design to illustrate major intellectual concepts and principles?
- Are the culturally diverse content, examples and experiences included comparable in kind, significance, magnitude and function to those selected from mainstream culture?
- Are the suggested methods for teaching content and skills and the proposed student learning activities responsive to the learning styles and preferences of different students?
- Do the evaluation techniques allow different ways for students to demonstrate their achievement? Are these sensitive to ethnic and cultural diversity?
- Will the proposed learning activities continually stimulate and interest different kinds of students?
- How do the content and learning activities affirm the cultures of diverse students?
- Will the self-esteem and confidence of diverse learners be improved by the curriculum methods and materials? (Gay, 1988)

These lists should be considered both as the curriculum is being written and after its implementation. Remember that evaluation is ongoing and should take place throughout the entire curricular process.

Maintaining and Modifying the Program

It is not enough to merely develop and implement curricula. If a program is to remain successful it must be fine tuned, revised, maintained and updated (Ames et al., 1992). Assessment is the first step to modification. All those involved (e.g., teachers, students, parents, administrators) should informally evaluate the process throughout.

Formal curriculum revision should be scheduled by the administration and occur at the very least annually. Administrators must also take responsibility for updating teachers and providing the budget to update materials as well.

Conclusions

Schools have always been a focal point of debate within the American culture. What should be taught, how should instruction be organized, what constitutes acceptable curriculum, and how should teachers be prepared? These questions have permeated education for decades. Health, however, is just now beginning to be realized as necessary for the achievement of education's overall goals.

Health education has always been interested in the uniqueness of individuals. It is only recently that education in general is beginning to look at the need to address individual differences. Therefore, health educators have the unique opportunity to be leaders in multicultural education.

We must begin by making our health education curricula culturally relevant. As depicted in the Multicultural Health Education Model, we must address diversity throughout all content areas to enable them as pieces of a puzzle to fit together to create a diverse yet cohesive understanding beyond ourselves and our communities (Pahnos, 1991).

References

Airhihenbuwa, C. O. and O. Pineiro. 1988. Cross-cultural health education: A pedagogical challenge. *Journal of School Health* 59 (6): 240-242.

Ames, E. E., L. A. Trucano, J. C. Wan and M. H. Harris. 1992. *Designing school health curricula.* Dubuque, IA: Wm. C. Brown.

Banks, J. A. 1981. *Multicultural education: Theory and practice.* Boston, MA: Allyn and Bacon.

Banks, J. A. 1991. Multicultural education: For freedom's sake. *Educational Leadership* 49 (4): 32-36.

Banks and Banks. 1993. *Multicultural education: Issues and perspectives.* Boston: Allyn and Bacon.

Bateman, D. R. 1974. *The politics of curriculum.* In *Heightened consciousness, cultural revolution and curriculum theory,* ed. W. Pinar. Berkeley, CA: McCuthan Publishers.

Gay, G. 1988. Designing relevant curricula for diverse learners. *Education and Urban Society* 2 (4): 327-340.

Matiella, A. C. 1991. *Positively different: Creating a bias-free environment for young children.* Santa Cruz, CA: ETR Associates.

Pahnos, M. L. 1991. Health educators as leaders in multicultural education. *The Reporter* 65 (1): 12.

Pahnos, M. L. 1992. The continuing challenge of multicultural health education. *Journal of School Health* 62 (1): 24-26.

Pahnos, M. L. and K. L. Butt. 1992. Ethnocentrism—A universal pride in one's ethnic background: Its impact on teaching and learning. *Education* 113:118-120.

Pollock, M. 1987. *Planning and implementing health education in schools.* Mountain View, CA: Mayfield Publishing Company.

Redican, K., Olsen, L. and C. Baffi. 1993. *Organization of school health programs.* Carmel, IN: WCB Brown and Benchmark.

Multicultural Relevancy in Instruction

Chapter 8

Empowerment Education Applied to Youth

Nina Wallerstein, DrPH

I n the past decade, the term "empowerment" has captured the imagination of people in public health, government and human services. Casual use of the term, however, has led to a wide disparity in definition, and a lack of clarity on the impact of "empowerment" on people's health, especially for youth.

This chapter presents a broad definition of community empowerment that embeds individuals in their social context. An empowerment educational methodology for people working with youth is described, with a case study of an adolescent alcohol use prevention program that illustrates the educational approach in practice.

In public health, empowerment has been largely defined by its opposite—powerlessness. Although powerlessness is recognized as having both a subjective and objective dimension (Seeman, 1959; Gaventa, 1980; Albee, 1981), the definition of empowerment most commonly used focuses on changing how people feel about themselves, treating individuals as separate from their social context. Many have adopted the empowerment rhetoric to promote a conservative agenda, blaming individuals for not having skills or motivation to rise out of powerlessness (Ryan, 1976).

A broader definition of empowerment proposes that people gain control of their own lives in the context of participating with others to change their social and political realities (Rappaport, 1987; Zimmerman and Rappaport, 1988). Community empowerment becomes a multilevel construct, with individual transformation occurring within the context of organizational, community and societal change. The goals of an empowerment social action process, therefore, are individual and community capacity building, control over life decisions, equity of resources, and improved quality of life (Wallerstein, 1992).

This community empowerment approach is particularly relevant for the increasing numbers of U.S. youth, who, for reasons of poverty, minority status, limited job opportunities, parent unemployment, discrimination or fear of the future, are at high risk. Youth today face the highest proportion of deaths from trauma, violence and motor vehicle crashes (often related to substance use) than any other age group. Minority youth are especially affected; they constitute 80 percent of all high school dropouts. Today, one in five children live in poverty, with Black and Hispanic children two to three times more likely than White children to be below the poverty level (Kids Count, 1992).

Despite the numbers of children subjected to poverty and violence, the dominant society continues to promote myths of equal opportunity and achievement of success through consumption. Young people are particularly vulnerable to the glamorous allure of advertising; the alcohol industry alone spends a billion dollars per year in advertising, with another billion for sponsorship of family events, such as rodeos, motor car racing and state fairs. While many youth express anger at the discrepancies between myth and reality, others blame themselves for their lack of opportunities and develop low self-esteem and feelings of powerlessness.

Knowing this about the alarming situations that youth face in their daily lives, I pose a critical question: How do we—as health specialists, educators, youth and human service workers—effectively address youth's social contexts which can vary considerably depending on ethnicity, culture, social class and gender? Equally important, how do we draw on the personal and cultural strengths of youth that can promote resiliency and growth for individuals and communities?

Unfortunately, prevailing youth programs such as job training, substance use prevention or drop-out prevention often use an individual definition of empowerment. These programs seek to promote self-esteem, self-efficacy, and improved competencies or life skills, which enable youth to better "function" in society.

The problems with competency or individual skill-building approaches are many. First, although youth benefit from learning a specific skill, such as how to fill out employment applications, many already know how to *function* quite well enough to survive in their worlds; in fact, they may have much to teach us about survival. Second, teaching functional skills often means teaching youth to fit into a prescribed role without questioning. For example, in job training programs students are often taught to respond to a supervisor's orders, but not to negotiate their rights.

Most important, education that exists in a vacuum, separate from life's pressures and complexities, only reinforces feelings of helplessness and inadequacy. Imagine a typical health lesson that teaches kids to resist peer pressure to take drugs. On the one hand, this practice is essential for behavior change and should be integral to any curriculum. Taken alone, however, this lesson ignores the reality that many youth face: the status or money they can earn from drugs. It also ignores the fears of youth that in saying "no" to their friends they will lose the all-important peer group that enables their development into adulthood. Without an opportunity to explore the underlying emotional, social or structural issues, youth may feel bored, patronized or, at worst, more powerless in their lives. In educational or community settings, these underlying issues can be thought of as "hidden voices," which can either block learning, or, if they become a central focus, can unleash learning and motivation to change.

Paulo Freire's Philosophy

An alternative approach to individual skill-building education—called popular or empowerment education—starts from these hidden voices or key issues in young people's lives. Through dialogue about these issues, youth are empowered to take an active social and political role in their communities. Inspired by Brazilian educator Paulo Freire, empowerment education involves people in group efforts to identify their own problems, to critically analyze the cultural and socioeconomic roots of the problems, and to develop strategies to effect positive changes in their lives and in their communities. In an alcohol use prevention program, for example, the goals of empowering education could include skill development and healthy behaviors, but would extend far beyond creating alcohol-free parties or drug-free ghettos. Community empowerment education would aim to foster healthy individuals in the context of creating healthy communities, such as involving youth in ridding neighborhoods of advertising targeted at minorities, or promoting economic development for young people.

Freire originally developed his ideas through highly successful literacy programs for slumdwellers in Brazil. Choosing emotionally and socially charged ("generative") words and pictures of students' problems, he generated discussion on how to improve their lives. In six weeks, people gained the literacy skills to vote and participate in the political process (Freire, 1970; Freire, 1973). In the last three decades, Freire's educational ideas have been a catalyst for worldwide programs in literacy (Fiore and Elsasser, 1992; Elsasser and John-Steiner, 1977); English as a second language (Wallerstein, 1983; Auerbach and Wallerstein, 1987); health education (Minkler, 1985; Werner and Bower, 1982; Wallerstein and Bernstein, 1988; Magaña and Ferreira-Pinto, 1992; Bialik-Gilad et al., 1991; Carpio-Cedraro et al., 1992; Labonte, 1992); worker health and safety (Wallerstein and Weinger, 1992); youth programs (Reed, 1981; Alschuler, 1980); college courses (Shor, 1980; Shor, 1987); and community development (Hope, Timmel and Hodzi, 1984; Barndt, 1989).

Freire's central premise is that education is never neutral, never value-free. In class or community settings, young people bring with them their life pressures and future expectations. In this context, Freire asks: Who does education serve and for what purpose? Does education prepare people to be objects of learning and to accept their place within the status quo, or does it liberate people to question the critical issues of the day and challenge the forces that keep them passive? Freire suggests that the hidden agenda for most learning experiences is the teaching of attitudes and behaviors of the dominant society, a practice which ignores the traditions of those on the outside—the ethnic minorities, youth and other disenfranchised peoples. This agenda is reinforced through traditional hierarchies where the teacher often represents one culture (if not ethnicity, then that of expertise or class), and the students represent another.

To equalize the hierarchical relationships and to equally value all cultures, Freire proposes a co-learner approach. Instead of treating students as empty vessels to be filled by teachers' knowledge, students become subjects of their own learning, using their life experiences, cultures and concerns as the starting point. Through *dialogue*, everyone—teacher and students—participates as co-learners to understand and create a jointly constructed reality.

The goal of group dialogue is critical thinking or posing problems in such a way as to uncover root causes of one's place in society—the socioeconomic, political, cultural and historical context of personal lives, and one's role in making changes. Critical thinking continues beyond perception and understanding, towards the *actions* that people can take to gain control over their lives.

In the United States, one of the most powerful applications of empowerment education is the Highlander Education and Research Center in Tennessee. Since the 1930s, Highlander has brought people together in residential workshops to tackle the problems of union organizing, literacy, citizenship, civil rights, strip mining, community development and youth leadership (Adams, 1975). Like Freire, Highlander focuses on the participatory group process of people sharing their lives, an analysis of political situations, and leadership development. To its founder Myles Horton, learning how to think and act on solving problems, or becoming "competent citizens," is primary.

Community organizing, in the Alinsky tradition, stresses action over reflection, contributing skills for societal change, such as choosing winnable goals, using confrontational tactics, and building "power" coalitions (Alinsky, 1971; Staples, 1984). Despite the different emphases of community organizing and popular education, all three traditions (from Freire, Horton and Alinsky) share common principles: starting from people's deeply felt concerns, moving from individual to collective action, shifting power into the hands of the previously disempowered, and developing strategies that can create actual change as well as expand the numbers of people involved in organizing.

Freire's Educational Methods

To transform community empowerment education theory into program development, Freire offers a three-stage method. The first step is listening for the key issues and emotional concerns (the "hidden voices") expressed by the youth. The second step is promoting participatory dialogue about these concerns. The third step is taking action about the concerns that are discussed. This final step is not an end point, but only part of the continuous cycle of action and reflection. After one action, students return to dialogue to reflect on their successes and failures, to re-listen for the key issues raised by the action, and to strategize new directions for actions. True knowledge evolves from the interaction of reflection and action (or *praxis*) to transform the social conditions.

Listening is key for several reasons. First, it enables the professional to solicit the hidden voices: the motivations and barriers to the learning process. Second, it enables the curriculum—in whatever content area—to emerge from the participants themselves, their life experiences, their cultural traditions, their interpretation of how they are in the world. If the curriculum is already prescribed, systematic listening will enable the educator or youth worker to place the existing lessons into an appropriate personal and cultural context. Third, listening builds genuine partnership and relationships between professionals and young people. Youth can be truly regarded as resources if their feelings, ideas and concerns form the basis of the program. The listening can be a shared exercise if youth are asked to participate in planning from the beginning, so they can discover key issues among themselves.

Once the hidden voices and key issues are uncovered, Freire

proposes creating discussion objects called "codes" (from the Portuguese codificaçao) or "triggers" because their purpose is to trigger dialogue. A trigger is a concrete physical representation of an identified issue in any form: a roleplay, story, slide or series of slides, short video (preferably five to ten minutes), photograph, song, rap, etc. Each trigger re-presents the participants' reality back to them and allows people to project their emotional, social and cultural responses in a focused fashion. Triggers are more than teaching aids about information. Their purpose is to generate critical thinking and actions about problems central to people's lives.

Take for example, a trigger about youth:

Ray: "Hey please, don't do that. Give me a break. I didn't see your flashing red light."

Police Officer: "I'm sorry. The law's the law. The sign says, 'No turn on red light,' outside the hospital. Sign here, please."

Ray: "No way. I'm not signing anything. I don't have a job. I can't pay the ticket. Can't you give me a break this time?"

Police: "What are you punks doing on this side of town anyway? Do you have a reason to be here? Let me see your car registration and insurance."

Ray: "Yeah, I have car insurance. I have a license too. And don't tell us where we can be. We can be in any part of town we want to."

Police: "Yeah, yeah, you still have to sign here saying you received this ticket. And I don't care where you want to be. Just get out of here and don't make any more trouble."

This roleplay could be used in a variety of settings: a life-skills class to discuss legal rights; a gang prevention program to discuss conflict mediation; a health class looking at the relationship between community systems and people.

Although triggers present open-ended situations, critical thinking does not occur spontaneously. Facilitators provide group leadership by using an inductive questioning strategy that moves discussion from the concrete and personal level to the social analysis and action stage.

Take for example the trigger presented above. To lead the discussion, the inductive questioning steps can best be remembered through the acronym SHOWED (Shaffer 1983). Step one and two elicit a concrete description of the trigger. In step one, the facilitator asks, what do you "See" in this dialogue? What is each person saying? The second series of questions focuses on what's really "Happening" here as the problem. How does each person, Ray and the police officer, feel about this situation? How do you think Ray feels about police officers? How do you think the police officer feels about teenagers? (Feeling questions can bring out the multiple perspectives of problems.)

In step three, the facilitator asks people to personalize the trigger, to see how the problem relates to "Our" lives. Is this a realistic situation? Do you know anyone who was treated this way by a police officer? What happened? How was it different? the same? Are there places where teenagers cruise in town? (It is better to ask about others and allow people to volunteer their own stories.)

In step four, the facilitator deepens the dialogue to an analytic level, asking "Why" there is a problem (on a cultural, social or historical level). Why was the teenager defensive? Why did the police officer think teenagers cause trouble? Are there cultural or racial issues here in the misunderstanding? What are the reasons that people assume there are appropriate areas of town for others?

What are the problems or benefits to teenage cruising? Is there a history to the problems?

The next two steps are the goal of the problem-posing process as they take the group towards actions. *E* stands for "Evaluation" and "Empowerment." What have we learned so far about the issues? Now that we better understand some aspect of the problems, how can we feel empowered to act for change?

Finally, what can we "Do" to solve the problem or choose strategies for action? How could each person in this dialogue have acted differently? What can we do to improve relations between police and youth in our community? How can we get involved? What steps can we take now to begin a process of change?

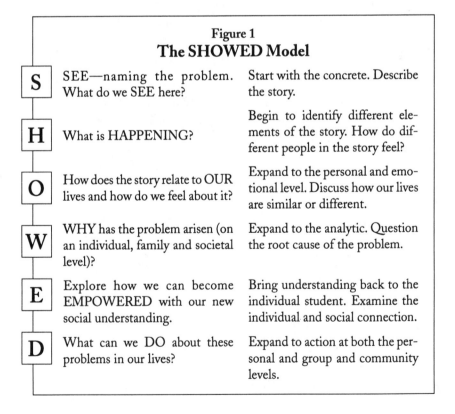

Figure 1
The SHOWED Model

S	SEE—naming the problem. What do we SEE here?	Start with the concrete. Describe the story.
H	What is HAPPENING?	Begin to identify different elements of the story. How do different people in the story feel?
O	How does the story relate to OUR lives and how do we feel about it?	Expand to the personal and emotional level. Discuss how our lives are similar or different.
W	WHY has the problem arisen (on an individual, family and societal level)?	Expand to the analytic. Question the root cause of the problem.
E	Explore how we can become EMPOWERED with our new social understanding.	Bring understanding back to the individual student. Examine the individual and social connection.
D	What can we DO about these problems in our lives?	Expand to action at both the personal and group and community levels.

The SHOWED acronym is one tool to promote a Freirian process of genuine listening and action. Although the steps are useful, true dialogue is not linear, but moves back and forth between steps, as participants place their personal experience into the social reality. In simpler terms, a Freirian dialogue is an interaction between two processes: understanding oneself in one's societal context (the "Our" and "Why" levels of SHOWED); and understanding the issues through a constant interaction of discussion and action (see Figure 2).

For example, after discussing the above trigger, youth could decide to research the relationship in their own communities between police and youth. This investigative action would stimulate greater dialogue and new understandings that could lead to further actions. Most important, it could lead the youth to understand the significance of reflection on a continuous basis, so they learn how to examine their own values and their own choices, and to acknowledge the consequences of their actions.

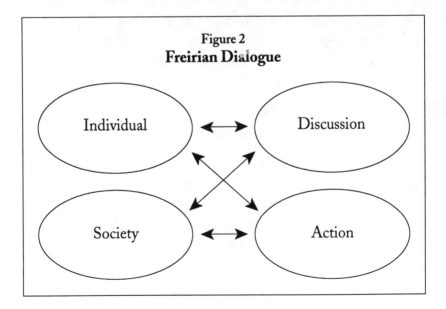

Figure 2
Freirian Dialogue

As seen through the dialogue questions, action emerges as the goal of critical thinking. Because of the possible multiplicity of targets for change, it is deceptive to consider this process problem-*solving*. As community organizers know, change best occurs when people choose short-term winnable goals which build the belief they can make a difference and which can alter the balance of power, (i.e., after this action, the youth group becomes a recognized force in the community).

Initial actions for youth are often informational or based on accepted educational activities. Young people may approach authorities for assistance, gather information for a photo display about their community, or conduct a contest. As they evaluate and celebrate the successes of their actions, the youth will identify what they've gained and what they have been unable to attain through the particular action. Instead of becoming frustrated with the futility of attempting to solve the problem, the celebration of success combined with the reflection on limitations nourishes people to choose the next action that may bring them closer to real community change. The process of empowerment therefore is called problem-*posing*, recognizing the complexity and long-term nature of individual and community change.

Curriculum Development with a Freirian Approach

As health practitioners, it may be difficult to imagine implementing this approach in practice. Curriculum is often prescribed. Categorical funding may restrict program objectives to specific topics. Therefore listening for people's hidden voices and concerns cannot be totally open. True community organizing, directed by the participants, cannot totally occur. In these cases, a Freirian approach can still contribute to ensuring that the program meets people's needs: in adopting as much as possible a participatory approach in the initial planning phase; in working with the youth as resources and decision-makers; in the use of triggers; in the role of the facilitator in promoting dialogue; and in having broadened goals which include cultural and social as well as behavioral changes.

In planning curricula or programs, educators usually develop objectives for information or behavior change. To apply Freire's philosophy, two other approaches need to be taken: adding social action and emotion-based objectives (Weinger and Wallerstein, 1990); and incorporating within each objective the dialogical framework of personal sharing, analytic understanding, and action planning (Arnold et al., n.d.).

Social action objectives will evolve in the course of addressing a community problem, but they can also be considered at the outset. Providing opportunities for youth to help others, for example, will help them develop belief and experience in social responsibility.

Emotion-based objectives are identified through the listening for hidden voices: What are people's fears, angers, attitudes about the problem, and desires for change? Because emotions can block or release learning, they need to be addressed in the beginning (and throughout) any program. The mechanism for uncovering emotions is the trigger which codifies the issues into a physical form to be used in the curriculum. Even with pre-existing curricula, triggers that portray the emotional and social context can be added to initiate the various curricular lessons throughout any program.

To create a roleplay or story trigger, the following steps may be useful:

1. Identify a key concern or issue that is a familiar daily problem to the participants.
2. Imagine the possible hidden voices or conflicting thoughts that people have about this situation.

3. Develop characters to reflect these voices.
4. Sketch out a dialogue or story that remains open-ended, with many sides portrayed.
5. Be sure to avoid putting a solution into the trigger. The strategies for resolving the problem should come from the group dialogue.

In visual triggers, such as slides or photographs, it is helpful to present people and to juxtapose images so that different voices can be drawn out in discussion.

The Role of the Facilitator

The role of the facilitator in Freirian dialogue differs from being a group discussion leader in a variety of ways. In Freirian dialogue, facilitators encourage genuine exchange of life experiences based on trust and listening, yet they do more than elicit and synthesize different points of view. In this approach, facilitators draw out students' strengths by first asking students to share their values, their traditions and their experiences. As the dialogue continues, facilitators challenge students to think critically about themselves and about societal forces and people's roles in social change. They encourage the group to determine their own actions for initiating the desired change.

To accomplish critical thinking, facilitators must walk a fine line between directing the dialogue to ensure all levels of thinking are reached, and listening carefully to uncover the group's issues. This means preparing questions in advance for each level of the SHOWED model, yet being willing to follow a new direction that may emerge in the dialogue. In the problem-posing dialogue, facilitators often find it difficult to ask analytic or "why" questions. Dialogue can easily jump from the personal story to the action stage. The analysis stage may be difficult for youth because of variations in their abstract thinking capabilities. Critical thinking, however, is central to preventing participants from becoming overwhelmed with their own personal stories. Often people may recognize the problems of poverty or historical discrimination, yet still feel isolated and blame themselves for their inability to transcend their environment.

An important and relatively unexplored aspect of Freirian facilitation concerns the power dynamics between the facilitator and students. Relationships of dominant and subordinate can be a result of school structural hierarchies, perceptions of facilitator expertise versus students' lack of knowledge, and facilitators who come from the dominant culture versus students who may be people of color or be otherwise in a marginal position. Co-learner relationships are neither inevitable, nor easily created. Facilitators who do not recognize the privilege that comes with their position may reinforce feelings of powerlessness and inadvertently perpetuate institutional racism or student silence (Pinderhughes, 1990). With that privilege therefore comes responsibility to unveil the power dynamics; to analyze race, gender or class dynamics in the classroom; and to be an advocate for students so that they can establish a genuine relationship as co-learners. Only by challenging power dynamics can facilitators "let go" of control over the direction of the group. The group actions that emerge then will not be imposed by the facilitator, but will be the result of democratic decision making.

The ability to work through conflicts and to allow emotions to surface in a relatively safe environment become important features of Freirian facilitation. If educators truly start from people's real issues, whether within the classroom or from the outside, then emotions will surface—past and present hurts, anger, or feelings of relief at finally being valued. Though facilitators may need to redirect emotions at times or talk after the session with someone who becomes upset, the emotions are also a necessary part of the change process. People's emotional responses are key to initiating change, building empathy with others, and maintaining motivation both for community-level change and for profound self-transformation.

Ultimately, the facilitator must perform a number of roles:

- Encourage a sharing of *everyone's* personal story, so people can see they are not alone.
- Be willing to address the emotional impact of discussing real issues.
- Listen and "name" the problem, for everyone to consider as equals.
- Ask how and why people's stories fit into a social and cultural context.
- Challenge power relationships within the classroom.

Placing youth stories into a social context can lead to the essential empowerment step of youth taking responsibility for doing something to challenge the negative forces in their environments, rather than remaining victims. Although people may be quick to identify actions, facilitators need to insist that the results of actions are evaluated and new actions planned. Evaluations nurture the idea of long-term change, based on a continuous cycle of reflection and action, and the need for supportive communities as part of organizing.

Evaluation of Empowerment Education

Though a large and diverse literature points to the association between empowerment and health outcomes (Wallerstein, 1992), evaluation of community empowerment programs is a complex undertaking. Clearly, empowerment can never be measured solely as an individual or personality variable. As discussed, changes may occur on the individual, organizational and community level. Yet individuals do become transformed as they participate in creating community change. Youth may change their perception of self-worth or their belief in their ability to take action, which replaces perceived powerlessness. Measures for these changes could include the construct psychological empowerment, which contains a number of interconnected social and intrapsychic variables, such as self-efficacy to take action, willingness to participate, and belief in group action (Zimmerman, 1990). Other important individual variables are empathy, critical thinking abilities, and outcome expectancies such as the belief that one's action makes a difference.

In addition to individual variables, a community empowerment program may produce organizational and community-setting change. Variables to measure could include improved social support and community bonding in a group of youth and improved community competence around youth issues, such as increased responsiveness to youth in a broad community coalition (Eng, 1992). More subtle impacts also could be noted, such as changes in cultural traditions of girls' participation in decision-making capacities. Ultimately, it is crucial to identify whether groups are becoming empowered to exert greater influence on larger entities, which may produce actual improvements in health or environmental conditions. These improvements as a result of advocacy pressures could be changes in policy, such as prohibiting tobacco sales to minors; changes in health-damaging economic development plans, such as preventing the placement of a toxic waste dump near a poor community; or changes in the political system, such as new county commissioners who are more responsive to youth issues and youth membership on county task forces.

In these variables, empowerment clearly is an interaction

between both process and outcome. As a process of involving others, empowerment means developing political efficacies, commitment and critical thinking that can lead to actual outcome changes. Though possible outcomes have been presented, a fixed state of an empowered individual or community is problematic. First of all, empowerment, as defined here, requires a bonding and commitment to others, and therefore individuals cannot be portrayed as "empowered" in isolation. Secondly, political reality is fluid. A community that may be successful in exercising its rights in one situation may be disempowered in another.

In sum, empowerment as a process and outcome may require measurement of changes on multiple levels, but also qualitative investigation into the context of change, through case study or ethnographic research. This may involve assessing the role of praxis within empowerment education, whether individuals are developing the reflective capability to judge their situations and make appropriate decisions on actions. Participatory research best lends itself to constant reflection on practice as youth or other members of the community become involved in planning and implementing the evaluation (Fals-Borda and Rahman, 1991; Tandon, 1989; McTaggart, 1991).

Alcohol and Substance Abuse Prevention Program

An example of a community health program that has adapted Freire's philosophy and methodology is the adolescent Alcohol and Substance Abuse Prevention program (ASAP), alternatively called the Adolescent Social Action Program (Wallerstein and Bernstein, 1988). ASAP aims to reduce excess morbidity and mortality among middle and high school students from high-risk, low-income, multiethnic communities. Sponsored since 1982 by the University of New Mexico School of Medicine, ASAP seeks to empower youth to make healthier choices in their own lives and, as community members, to play an active political role in their communities and society.

ASAP brings in small groups of teenage volunteer students from communities throughout New Mexico to talk with patients and families in several hospitals, and with residents in county detention centers who have suffered the consequences of alcohol and drug abuse, interpersonal violence, or unprotected sexual activity. ASAP emphasizes Freirian principles of experiential learning, dialogue, sharing their own lives and cultures, empathy, critical thinking and social action.

The groups are facilitated by university medical, nursing, education and counseling students who help direct the interviews and lead youth through a defined curriculum. The curriculum is based on current models of adolescent health promotion, such as cognitive-behavioral, resistance to social influence, and life skills approaches (Hansen et al., 1988; Shope et al., 1992; Perry, 1986), and the protection-motivation theory of behavior change (Rippetoe and Rogers, 1987; Rogers, 1983). Protection-motivation theory states that motivation comes from a combination of personalizing the consequences of unhealthy behaviors and developing the self-efficacies or coping skills to change one's behavior.

During their visits to the hospital and jail, the youth receive training in coping skills, communication and decision making, peer teaching techniques, and analysis of media and social policies that influence consumption, such as New Mexico's drive-up liquor windows. After four visits to the facilities, youth are trained back at their school sites as peer educators to spread the program to younger youth. The peer approach reinforces students' self-efficacies related to their own behaviors, fosters social responsibility, and facilitates bicultural competence (Perry, 1987; Klepp et al., 1986; Botvin et al., 1988).

By adopting the Freirian perspective, ASAP distinguishes itself from "Scared Straight" programs. Although initially the hospital and jail environment may be frightening or cause anxiety, the emphasis on dialogue shifts the focus to the youths' feelings, their world view, and their solutions to the problems they face in their communities. The coping skills curriculum linked with additional training in peer education techniques back at their school sites, assists the students in becoming leaders in their schools and communities. The action stage of ASAP has included many student projects, such as peer teaching with students in lower grades, developing videos on their own communities, writing a rap song to play on a local radio station, or testifying at tribal council meetings.

The discussion triggers and the problem-posing dialogue methodology form an important link between the ASAP hospital/jail experience, community outreach and youth empowerment. In the hospital, the patients and their life stories become the triggers for students to talk about their own lives. Outside the hospital, ASAP students lead peer discussions through several short video triggers developed by ASAP, or they create their own triggers about their own community situations. An additional classroom-based curriculum enables teachers and community professionals who don't have access to a hospital or jail setting to implement the dialogue methodology in their school systems.

Research on the program has pointed to increased awareness of the riskiness of drinking and driving among program participants after an eight-month follow-up as compared to a decrease in riskiness perception by the control group (Bernstein and Woodall, 1987); and increased self-efficacies for helping parents and friends (unpublished data). The pre- and posttest data collected on individuals and the participant observations of youth actions suggest that the program is having an effect on psychological empowerment variables, as well as community competence dimensions, such as the youths' ability to articulate themselves as political actors in their worlds.

In sum, the ASAP program incorporates Freire's underlying philosophy of personal and social transformation with youth who often experience societal inequalities, cultural conflicts or powerlessness. The educational problem-posing approach with triggers and dialogue helps people move beyond barriers to learning and involves them in a group process to change their lives as learners and as emerging teachers in their communities.

Conclusion

Empowerment education for change—personal, educational or socioeconomic—is an ongoing process that demands time and continued commitment. It demands a high level of self-reflection as health professionals and teachers to challenge our own assumptions, our own positions of privilege, and our own willingness to work in partnership with youth and with communities. While empowerment education does not automatically eliminate power relationships or structural inequities, this approach can encourage community decision making, community leadership and community transformation.

We must be "patiently impatient," Paulo Freire tells us, as we painstakingly move towards better quality of life and justice in our communities. Although change may evolve slowly, problem-posing can be a nurturing process as people explore visions and building community together as they work on problems.

References

Adams, F. 1975. *Unearthing seeds of fire: The idea of highlander.* Winston-Salem, NC: John Blair Press.

Albee, G. 1981. Politics, power, prevention, and social change. In *Prevention through political action and social change,* ed. J. Joffe and G. Albee, 5-25. University Press of New England, Hanover and London.

Alinsky, S. 1971. *Rules for radicals.* New York: Random House.

Alschuler, A. 1980. *School discipline: A socially literate solution.* New York: McGraw Hill.

Arnold, R., D. Barndt and B. Burke. n.d. *A new weave: Popular education in Canada and Central America.* Toronto, Canada: CVSO Development Education and the Ontario Institute for Studies in Education, Adult Education Department.

Auerbach, E., and N. Wallerstein. 1987. *ESL for action: Problem-posing at work* (teacher guide and student book). Reading, MA: Addison-Wesley.

Barndt, D. 1989. *Naming the moment: Political analysis for action.* Toronto, Canada: Jesuit Centre for Social Faith and Justice.

Bernstein, E., and W. G. Woodall. 1987. Changing perceptions of riskiness in drinking, drugs, and driving: An emergency department-based alcohol and substance abuse prevention program. *Annals of Emergency Medicine* 1350/67-1350/71.

Bialik-Gilad, R., R. Nagana and J. Ferreira-Pinto. 1991. Talking posters: A Freirean approach: The American Red Cross experience. *Border Health Special* 7 (1): 14-18.

Botvin, G. J., M. S. Moncher, M. A. Orlandi, J. Palleja, S. P. Schinke and R. F. Schilling. 1988. Preventing substance abuse among minority group adolescents: Applications of riskbased interventions. *Practice Applications* 4 (4): 1-16.

Carpio-Cedraro, F., A. De Carpio and L. Anderson. 1992. El programa "Comida para el Pensamiento": Un enfoque participativo en la prevención del sida. *Revista Latino Americana de Sicología* 24 (1/2): 137-156.

Elsasser, N., and V. John-Steiner. 1977. An interactionist approach to advancing literacy. *Harvard Education Review* 47 (3).

Eng, E. 1992. Community empowerment: The critical base. *Family and Community Health* 15 (1): 1-12.

Fals-Borda, O., and M. A. Rahman. 1991. *Action and knowledge.* New York: Apex Press.

Fiore, K., and N. Elsasser. 1992. Strangers no more: A liberatory literacy curriculum. *College English* 44 (2): 115-128.

Freire, P. 1970. *Pedagogy of the oppressed.* New York: Seabury Press.

Freire, P. 1973. *Education for critical consciousness.* New York: Seabury Press.

Gaventa, J. 1980. *Power and powerlessness.* Chicago, IL: University of Illinois Press.

Hansen, W. B., C. Johnson, B. Flay, J. Graham and J. Sobel. 1988. Affective and social influences approaches to the prevention of multiple substance abuse among seventh grade students: Results from Project SMART. *Preventive Medicine* 17:135-154.

Hope, A., S. Timmel and C. Hodzi. 1984. *Training for transformation: A handbook for community workers.* Vol. 1-3. Gweru, Zimbabwe: Mambo Press.

Kids Count Data Book. 1992. Washington, DC: Center for the Study of Social Policy.

Klepp, K. I., A. Halper and C. L. Perry. 1986. The efficacy of peer leaders in drug abuse prevention. *Journal of School Health* 56 (9): 407-411.

Labonte, R. 1992. Heart health inequalities in Canada: Models, theory and planning. *Health Promotion International* 7 (2): 119-128.

Magaña, J. R., and J. Ferreira-Pinto. 1992. Una pedagogia de concentración para la prevención del HIV/Sida. *Revista Latino Americana de Sicología* 24 (1/2): 97-108.

McTaggart, R. 1991. Principles for participatory action research. *Adult Education Quarterly* 41 (3): 168-187.

Minkler, M. 1985. Building supportive ties and sense of community among the inner-city elderly: The tenderloin outreach project. *Health Education Quarterly* 12 (4): 303-314.

Perry, C. 1986. Tobacco use among adolescents: Promising trends in prevention and cessation strategies. In *Behavioral Medicine: A Practical Handbook,* ed. T. Coates. New York: Wiley.

Perry, C. 1987. Results of prevention programs with adolescents. *Drug and Alcohol Dependence* 20:13-19.

Pinderhughes, D. 1990. *Understanding race ethnicity and power: The key to efficacy in clinical practice.* New York: The Free Press.

Rappaport, J. 1987. Terms of empowerment/examples of prevention: Toward a theory of community psychology. *American Journal of Community Psychology* 15 (2): 121-148.

Reed, D. 1981. *Education for building a people's movement.* Boston, MA: South End Press.

Rippetoe, P. A., and R. W. Rogers. 1987. Effects of components of protection-motivation theory on adaptive and maladaptive coping with a health threat. *Journal of Personality and Social Psychology* 52 (3): 596-604.

Rogers, R. 1983. Cognitive and physiological processes in fear appeals and attitude changes: A revised theory of protection motivation. In *Social psychophysiology: A source book,* ed. J. Cacioppo and R. Petty, 153-175. New York: The Guilford Press.

Ryan, W. 1976. *Blaming the victim.* Revised ed. New York: Vintage Books.

Seeman, M. 1959. On the meaning of alienation. *American Sociological Review* 24:783-791.

Shaffer, R. 1983. *Beyond the dispensary.* Nairobi, Kenya: Amref.

Shope, J. T., T. E. Dielman, A. Butchart, P. Campanelli and D. Kloska. 1992. An elementary school-based alcohol misuse prevention program: A follow-up evaluation. *Journal of Studies on Alcohol* 53 (2): 106-121.

Shor, I. 1980. *Critical teaching and everyday life.* Boston: South End Press.

Shor, I., ed. 1987. *Freire for the classroom: A sourcebook for liberatory teaching.* New Haven, CT: Boynton/Cook Publishers.

Staples, L. 1984. *Roots to power a manual for grassroots organizing.* New York: Praeger Publishing.

Tandon, R. 1989. *Movement towards democratization of knowledge.* New Delhi, India: Society for Participatory Research in Asia.

Wallerstein, N. 1983. *Language and culture in conflict: Problem posing in the ESL classroom.* Reading, MA: Addison-Wesley.

Wallerstein, N. 1992. Powerless, empowerment, and health: Implications for health promotion programs. *American Journal of Health Promotion* 6 (3): 197-205.

Wallerstein, N., and E. Bernstein. 1988. Empowerment education: Freire's ideas adapted to health education. *Health Education Quarterly* 15 (4): 379-394.

Wallerstein, N., and M. Weinger, eds. 1992. Empowerment approaches to worker health and safety education. *American Journal of Industrial Medicine* 22 (5).

Weinger, M., and N. Wallerstein. 1990. Education for action: An innovative approach to training hospital employees. In *Essentials of modern hospital safety,* ed. W. Charney and J. Schirmer, 321-342. Chelsea, MI: Lewis Publishers.

Werner, D., and B. Bower. 1982. *Helping health workers learn.* Palo Alto, CA: The Hesperian Foundation.

Zimmerman, M. 1990. Taking aim on empowerment research: On the distinction between individual and psychological conceptions. *American Journal of Community Psychology* 18 (1): 169-177.

Zimmerman, M., and J. Rapport. 1988. Citizen participation, perceived control and psychological empowerment. *American Journal of Community Psychology* 16 (5): 725-750.

Chapter 9

Student-Produced Health Education Materials

Rima E. Rudd, ScD,
Linda R. Comfort, RN, MPH,
Jeanne M. Mongillo, RNC, MPH,
and Linda M. Zani, RN

E ducators have long known that the most successful educational experiences are those that involve and engage the student. Experiential, active, participatory learning activities offer students opportunities to try out new skills, to shape and pace events to fit their learning needs, and to ground the topics and skills in the reality of their own lives. Albert Bandura (1986) notes that this approach builds self-efficacy. Paulo Freire (1968b) claims that such an approach is the bedrock of true education.

One mechanism for increasing learner participation in the educational experience is student involvement in the design and development of the learning materials. The learning materials that support the educational process often serve as the only tangible aspect of that experience. The materials production process can augment and reflect the key elements of the educational program and the production activities can offer a powerful learning intervention for those involved. Furthermore, learning materials developed by and credited to fellow students offer models of student efficacy and action for other readers.

This discussion highlights four case descriptions of student-generated materials. Each program took place within a school setting, one in a rural area and three in a major city. The health topics range from drug use (tobacco, alcohol and other drugs) to violence. In each case, however, learning materials were developed by the school children as part of an educational program to help students address important health-related topics. The focus of the discussion is on the participatory process, caveats and lessons learned. The descriptions of the process and key events are geared toward helping practitioners replicate such a program. Because the design of the activities in each of the cases was inspired by the concept of problem-posing education and modeled on a Freirean culture circle, the discussion begins with a brief examination of the Freirean pedagogy and methods.

Background: Freire's Process and Materials

Paulo Freire articulated and described a problem-posing approach to education which could serve to empower learners. "Problem-posing" education is action oriented and was offered in direct contrast to what Freire called "banking" education, a process that places the learners in a passive role—empty bank accounts to be filled with the wealth of teachers' knowledge. Problem-posing education, on the other hand, establishes a situation of equality, dialogue and mutual communication between students and teachers. This type of education, according to Freire, enables students to become reflective, self-conscious agents and critical thinkers capable of transforming the world.

Freire believes that the form of the learning materials is as important as the structure of the educational process (Brown, 1974). Freire's learning materials designed to lead participants through a process of discussion and discovery to "critical thinking." The materials he used consisted of a series of drawings that illustrated the distinction between culture and nature. These drawings were discussed within a culture circle (a group of learners with a facilitator who helped structure the discussion) and were meant to stimulate discussion, helping participants discover themselves as the makers of culture and agents of change. This was the start of the process Freire called "conscientização"—a process whereby participants are encouraged to analyze their own reality, become aware of the constraints put on their lives, and take action to transform their world (Brown, 1974).

Another set of materials offered depictions of generative themes that were used to further stimulate discussion and also teach the elements of literacy (Freire, 1968a). The materials were carefully crafted by Freire and his colleagues. Words describing important aspects of people's lives were compiled and the grouping of words was structured so that they would, in total, represent all the sounds of the language. These words were introduced first as drawings which helped learners describe some aspect of their lives, discuss problems and their causes, and consider possible action and solutions. The participants would then learn the letters and sounds of the words. Then the group would take action and meet again to reflect and to craft new action options. These activities constituted what Freire called "praxis"—a continuing cycle of reflection and action. Thus, Freire's materials supported an empowering process that allowed learners to define the content and the outcome of their own learning.

Participant-Developed Learning Materials

Freire's work has inspired many nationwide literacy programs, adult learning efforts, and innovative health education interventions. Many practitioners have sought to "translate" Freire's education process, and, as Minkler and Cox noted in 1980, often modified the methodology to fit their field needs. Two early modifications of Freire's work inspired the materials development cases discussed here.

First, a project implemented by the University of Massachusetts and the Ministry of Education in Ecuador experimented with additional forms of learning materials for the culture circle discussion. The Ecuador Project (Center for International Education, 1975) produced photonovels (called "fotonovelas" in Spanish), books which are formatted like comic books, tell a story, but contain photographs of people instead of cartoons. This format is used for popular literature in many countries in South and Central America. But, unlike commercial photonovels, those produced by the project used the learners and other local people as actors. Comings and Cain took this project one step further and explored the potential for learners, not the teachers or experts, to develop the materials. They facilitated the development of participant-designed photonovels with farmworkers for their own literacy classes and with community members in an environmental health program (Comings, Franz and Cain, 1981).

Photonovels: Depicting Generative Themes

Photonovels offer a fit with the tradition of Freire's materials because the stories draw on people's experiences, can illustrate important issues, and help readers focus on important themes. Learners focus on an issue or problem within the context of a drama which holds readers' attention and interest. In addition, the dialogue of the story, drawn directly from people's actual speech, provides reading material at relevant literacy levels (Roter et al., 1987). When the learners themselves can determine the content and the issues, decide on the action of the story, and give voice and shape to the characters, the materials may hold greater appeal and power for them and their peers than commercially developed materials might (Comings, 1979). Furthermore, learners of various ages can bring a wide variety of skills to the process and do not need sophisticated technological or artistic expertise.

Photonovel Production Process

Overall, student-produced photonovels can be developed through a very simple process. First, however, the facilitators must establish the guidelines of the program with all gatekeepers—school administrators, teachers and parents. Such support is critical for program implementation. Furthermore, facilitators and students must clarify constraints or limitations (including editorial and financial issues) and establish an atmosphere conducive to trust, sharing and exploration.

Ideally, students address issues of importance to them. When programs have predetermined topics (and health education programs frequently do), students should have the freedom to address their most important issues and be able to integrate their own concerns into the story. Students, as producers, should also have a voice regarding the use and distribution plans for their products. Needed materials (newsprint, paper, typewriter, cameras, film) must be available and printing options explored before the process begins. A checklist for each stage of the production process proves quite helpful. Figure 1 offers a sample of checklist items.

The production process can then get underway. Students need an opportunity to freely discuss the issue at hand. The story often begins with students identifying a main character or characters who, like themselves, face a problem. Generally, the story is simply based on an action or decision related to the issue. Next, students add characters, outline a story sequence, and begin to

---

Figure 1
Photonovel Production Checklist

Area of Concern	Sample Questions
Problem Posing	_____ Health issue of importance to participants is identified.
	_____ The message of the book is determined by participants.
Story Development	_____ Main character, problem/decision and outcome are determined.
	_____ Story sketch conveys the message participants determined.
Plot Sketch	_____ Each page is a complete scene.
	_____ The action within one page is kept to one setting.
	_____ The dialogue within each picture is fairly minimal.
First Layout	_____ The number and sequence of photographs is determined.
	_____ The person talking and the dialogue is set for each shot.
Production	_____ Actors and extras are chosen.
	_____ All props are identified and gathered.
	_____ All equipment is available.
Mock-up	_____ All pictures are chosen.
	_____ All headings and lead-ins are typed.
	_____ All elements of the book are in order.
	_____ Facing pages look good together.
Printing	_____ Paper, cover stock and ink selected.
	_____ Number of copies determined.

---

illustrate it with stick figures and a few simple words. A story board gives shape to the book and consists of a page by page sketch of the action illustrated with stick figures. Dialogue is then added. Frequently, a brief sentence can serve to offer transition where needed.

Finally, the book takes form with a photography session: participants, other students and adults become the "actors" in the story. Neighborhood scenes, if captured in a photonovel, reflect the world of the students. Indoor scenes can also be easily constructed. One project, for example, set up a hospital room in the school cafeteria with materials borrowed from a local health center. After the film is processed, pictures are then chosen and laid out on a story board, dialogue bubbles typed and pasted on, and a mock-up produced. There is ample opportunity at each stage to rewrite, recast and change the book. The final materials can take various forms: a bulletin board display, a photocopied and stapled booklet, a newspaper-like product, or a printed book. Clearly, costs are a consideration. Figure 2 provides a sample budget checklist to determine production costs.

School-Based Applications

There are more than 46 million students and 5 million faculty and staff each year in the 100,000 public and private elementary and secondary schools in this country. Schools provide the most systematic and efficient means available for reaching young children (McGinnis and DeGraw, 1991). These institutions can do more than any other single agency to help young people live longer, healthier lives (Allensworth and Kolbe, 1987). Clearly, school health programs have the potential to have a great impact on the health of children and the adults they will become. Students acquire knowledge, develop attitudes, learn new behaviors and

---

Figure 2
Sample Budget Checklist

This is a sample budget checklist to produce 100 booklets. Each booklet is approximately ten pages long, with three to four pictures on each page. Please note that some of the materials and services listed below can be obtained at low or no cost.

Equipment
    2 - 35mm cameras with flash   _____
    1 - Instant camera   _____

Film
    3 - Rolls black and white film (36 exposures)   _____
    4 - Packages instant film   _____

Film development   _____

Halftone conversions   _____

60 lb. standard white paper (11" x 17")   _____

Printing (including folding, collating and stapling)   _____

Miscellaneous materials/costs   _____
(This category can include paper products, student prizes
and end of the program celebration.)

---

skills as a result of effective school health programs. This knowledge and skill base enables individuals to make informed choices about behaviors that will affect their own health throughout their lives. In addition, as students enter adulthood, they take on responsibility for the health of their families and the health of their communities and can, with others, influence their environments and worksites. Thus, school-based programs can effect lasting change (McGinnis and DeGraw, 1991).

In spite of the development of creative health education models that have evolved during the past thirty years, evaluation studies have had difficulty documenting a clear correlation between program offerings and the desired behavior change sustained over time. As those individual and collective behaviors that pose a threat to health have become more widely studied, researchers have been finding multiple levels of complexity. Consequently, school-based health education programs have been expanding in scope to include information on the immediate as well as long-term physiological and social consequences of individual and institutional behaviors, an understanding of the social forces supportive of certain behaviors, and the development of analytic and social skills to affect the prevalence of those behaviors. In addition, many programs address issues of self-efficacy and social norms and are designed to help students enhance the development of personal and collective skills to resist social pressures as well as effect supportive environmental change (Flay, 1985).

Inspired by the Freirean pedagogy, Wallerstein and Bernstein call for an empowerment model for health education programs. This approach is defined as a social action process that promotes participation of people, organizations and communities in gaining control over their lives in the community and in the larger society (Wallerstein and Bernstein, 1988). The goal of an empowerment educational strategy is to develop a participatory model of health education that is learner directed and focuses on the group's ideas of what they believe to be important to them. As the group identifies areas of concern, they begin to develop strategies for solving the problem. As students work together, they acquire the skills and power to realize that they can make changes and gain control in their own lives as well as have some influence on others.

Participatory Materials Development: Four Cases

There are a variety of mechanisms for integrating this model into the classroom. The implementation of empowerment education programs in the schools, both public and private, can be exciting and challenging, offering new concepts and techniques to the students, the faculty and the administration. The four participatory materials development programs described here were designed to do just this.

The four cases are linked. The materials developed in the first case served as the guideline for the subsequent cases (Rudd, Kichen and Joslin, 1980). The facilitators for the programs in the second, third and fourth cases worked together, and, in each subsequent case, learned from and built on the previous experiences. Although all of the four "photonovels" profiled in this chapter followed the same basic process, each resulted in a unique experience. The case discussions offer descriptions of the process undertaken and articulation of the lessons learned.

Case 1: Smoking Prevention Materials

The first case, focused on smoking prevention among early adolescents, was designed to encourage the inclusion of effective smoking prevention programs in schools in a rural county of western Massachusetts. Of particular interest to the project director was the concept of a county technical high school developing the capability to produce low-cost, locally oriented materials for its students and for younger students in feeder schools. With the approval of school administration, the parent-teacher association, and the classroom teachers, project staff recruited ninth grade participants and worked with them in their English class.

Students were asked to work within pre-established parameters. The project had been funded by the Centers for Disease Control and Prevention to focus on smoking prevention and the project director had arranged for materials to be used in the technical school and also in selected elementary schools. Although students had the opportunity to include issues of interest to them in the design of their product, they did have to focus on smoking prevention. Thus, participation in the determination of the problem was limited; however, the structure of the production process was strongly influenced by the Freirean culture circle approach.

The ninth grade students identified a variety of positive and negative issues concerning cigarette smoking (a force field analysis), interviewed adults and peers about their decisions to smoke or not smoke, discussed their dilemmas, and began to develop a story that would illustrate their issues related to smoking. This process reflected an approximation of Freire's problem-posing elements:

- Analyze their reality. (smoking embedded in issues of early adolescence)
- Search for root causes. (the hard sell of advertisers, peer pressure and modeled adult behavior)
- Be aware of constraints. (the pros and cons of smoking)
- Develop a plan of action. (produce health education materials)

It is important to note, however, that the "action" seen as the production of an educational book in the form of a photonovel, was clearly predetermined and imposed from without. The students started from and did not determine this action plan.

As students struggled with developing one main storyline, it became clear that the girls and boys wanted to focus on very different issues. The girls and boys developed independent story lines and the class decided to track the two main characters (a girl and a boy) throughout the book and present the girl's story on one side of a page and the boy's on the other. The two characters were brought together during a party at the book's conclusion. The characters focused on those smoking-related issues of concern to the students: problems such as ash burns on clothing, the effort needed to practice smoking, barriers of cost, social pressures to be part of a group, and romantic constraints concerning smells; long-term health effects were of little or no importance. The format of the photonovel and the issues under discussion emerged from student needs and might not have been included in an adult "expert" production.

Students were the decision-makers throughout the production process (including the various processes of determining the story, writing the dialogue, sketching the action, setting up scenes, holding photography sessions, and preparing the final layout) and completed a twelve-page book titled *Decisions, Decisions.* Groups of other students contributed to the book by designing fact sheets and counter advertisements.

Overall, the product was enthusiastically received and the process well rated. Students planned for the high school distribution of the finished product, developed one of the evaluation instruments, and contributed to a teachers' guide for the use of the materials. The teachers' guide, however, was written by the project director with local school health educators. The photonovel served as the basis for lessons on smoking prevention for ninth graders conducted through the English and science classes. On the day of schoolwide distribution, reporters from the local newspaper and television news station covered the day's activities.

In addition, fifth graders from two neighboring schools also received copies of the photonovel in conjunction with a lesson on smoking prevention. This aspect of the program did not involve the student producers (although they helped design, enter and process the user evaluations). The program might well have been strengthened by bringing the producers into the classrooms of younger students. However, the fifth graders noted and liked the listing of the names and home towns of all the producers and the ninth graders received the results of the evaluations.

The project evaluation included an examination of health locus of control, intent to smoke and smoking behavior, as well as subjective assessments of the value of a participatory process, teacher ratings on student receptiveness and responsiveness, and user ratings on readability, relevancy and preference (Rudd and Kichen, 1980). While all of the health-related indicators were in a positive direction, analysis revealed no statistically significant change. Overall, the student and teacher ratings were quite high.

Although not discovered or acknowledged until the end, the boys had decided to use as the actor for their main character a young man well known to be a heavy smoker. These and other built-in jokes surely had an effect on the peer group reading the materials but did not appear to influence the overall enthusiastic reception granted to the book.

Teachers were encouraged to become part of the process and most were quite supportive and became actively involved. The materials were used in the classrooms as planned. However, without outside funding, support, and expertise, the materials production process was not repeated and additional products were not forthcoming. The facilitators of the three subsequent cases were attentive to the process, the limitations and the issues raised in this case.

Urban Programs

The three photonovel projects that followed were facilitated by public health nurses working for the School Health Program, Boston's Department of Health and Hospitals, Division of Public Health. The School Health Program is a community-based initiative providing health services/health education to school-age children, grades K through 8, who attend parochial/private schools in Boston. The 11,000 students and faculty are culturally and economically diverse, reflecting the neighborhood where each school is located.

Case 2: Alcohol Use Prevention

In the second case, the faculty and staff of an urban school requested an educational intervention addressing the excessive use of alcohol among eighth grade students attending that school. The health education literature on alcohol issues suggests that in virtually every class of thirty children, regardless of geographic area, socioeconomic level or academic achievements, about eight to ten students live with or have been seriously affected by family alcoholism. Furthermore, research findings indicate that children of alcoholics have four times greater risk of developing the disease (CASPAR, 1987). Thus, it was estimated that at least 12 students in the class of 42 students at this urban school would likely come from a home in which one or both parents were problem drinkers.

A surprisingly large percentage (80 percent) of the students admitted to using alcohol at least once a month with friends to get drunk. Previous alcohol education efforts in the school had consisted of the administration of a ten-lesson curriculum, delivered sequentially over a two-week period. Frustrations among school staff grew, however, when excess alcohol use remained problematic among students in spite of this ongoing program. While students were able to assimilate knowledge about alcohol from this structured approach, they were unable to follow through and make the changes in their own behavior which would result in decrease or non-use of this substance. The school administration and faculty were open to new possibilities.

As more discussion took place about the health problem, it

became clear to staff that excessive alcohol use among students and the issues that led to that behavior were more deeply rooted than were being addressed in the existing program. The facilitators selected an empowerment theoretical framework which provided an avenue of self-awareness and self-direction for the students. The empowerment model enables students to critically analyze the problem themselves, strategize, and offer potential solutions. Thus, the facilitators suggested an intervention that would provide a collaborative learning experience which the students could personalize. They postulated that through this Freirean approach, students would develop the skills necessary to learn to work together as a group, identify a problem that was adversely affecting their lives, and formulate a solution. Furthermore, through the confidence gained from this experience, students would begin to relate proactively in decision making leading to positive behavior change. The materials developed in the first case provided the foundation for this work. Students were interested in producing a book and in exploring the issues of alcohol use.

As in the first case, eighth grade students wrote and produced the photonovel with the eventual goal of using it as a teaching tool for students in the lower grades. Three facilitators helped guide the students through the overall process. Although participation in the project was voluntary, all 42 students chose to take part. The group met weekly and the project was completed over the course of the school year.

Facilitators and students began by creating their version of the "culture circle." It was in this forum that the health problem was discussed informally. Students were asked to relate the problem to their own lives, and, without fear of censorship, began to expound upon how their personal experiences with alcohol might be used to convey important information about the topic to their target population through the photonovel. This idea is central to Freire's premise that education is not neutral, that it starts from the experiences of people and either reinforces or challenges the existing social forces that keep them passive.

Students were subsequently asked to brainstorm the list of committees they thought would need to be formed to complete the task of photonovel production from start to finish. They then self-selected their committee assignment by area of interest. Once the committees were formed, facilitators spent time working with each group to help them delineate the details of the production. Unlike the first case where there was an external source of funds, no funding was available for the materials production. Consequently, students were also faced with the task of raising money to cover expenses. This resulted in an expansion of student participation as they were involved in all aspects of production, from fundraising to storyline development and final layout. They also portrayed the actors and actresses in the book, wrote the dialogue, and developed a teachers' guide for classroom use. Each week, representatives of the various committees would make brief verbal reports to their fellow students about the work that was being accomplished in their group.

Throughout the entire production, the role of the facilitator was that of a guide, helping to direct the project and not dictating or attempting to control the process. Wallerstein identifies this role of the Freirean educator as problem posing instead of problem solving. This establishes the leader or facilitator as a probing, critical inquirer rather than as a mechanical answer-giver with a present syllabus (Shorr, 1987). Facilitators also took responsibility for communicating production events to other faculty and school personnel through brief written updates every two weeks. Parental involvement was encouraged and the facilitators sent notes to parents to convey information about the production and also to communicate positive attributes about their child's contribution to the photonovel. These notes home provided a positive incentive and were welcomed by students, many of whom had never had a teacher write a positive note home to a parent.

As production progressed, students began to demonstrate more independence with the process. They wanted to be sure the storyline reflected their reality and returned to add and change elements. The major theme they chose was drinking and driving. Since this was a class of eighth-grade students, none of whom were of legal driving age, the facilitators at first could not understand their logic in choosing this particular theme as the major focus of their work. Students explained that while they themselves could not drive, many had older friends who were driving. When they would gather in the park to drink, these students would often be faced with the dilemma of whether or not to accept a ride. The main character faced this choice, one which was reality-based and personal.

Trust in the group process grew during the development of the storyline, and students felt more comfortable discussing their feelings, attitudes and beliefs about the problem without fear of judgment. For many students the collaborative learning process was a new phenomenon. Students needed to acquire the skill of negotiation when working with their peers, especially around issues concerning the storyline and dialogue development. For some students who were dealing with issues around alcohol at home, the topic proved to be anxiety-provoking and resulted in some acting-out behavior. The facilitators had to occasionally intervene and provide counseling in a nonpunitive manner.

The photonovel, *Friend or Foe,* was completed in May. Students held a variety of fundraising events including bake sales to cover their expenses. The original plan called for students at a local technical high school to print the booklet but, due to last minute fiscal constraints, this school was unable to fulfill the contract and a professional printer was chosen.

Students who produced the book were able to feel that their ideas and solutions were important and also that they had gained some control over their learning process. They acquired group skills, strategizing techniques, problem-solving abilities and the power of community organizing experience. They were able to view the educator in a new role, one as advisor and guide who validated and valued the personal experiences that students brought to the project. Younger students who received the book for classroom use could relate to the upper-grade actors and actresses in the photonovel as people like themselves who shared common problems and concerns.

Evaluation results supported the fact that the majority of students enjoyed working on their booklet a great deal and were satisfied with the way it appeared. Many also said it was better than other materials they had read concerning the topic. In addition, a majority of students felt they had personally made an important contribution to the development of the photonovel. Overall, students directed all phases of production and the result was a student-produced health education booklet which is personalized and yet relevant to many other groups.

Case 3: Violence Prevention

The photonovel produced in the third case focused on issues of violence. This topic was chosen by students in a school located in a part of the city where violence, in many forms, is pervasive. Gang violence was a major concern of these students. The facilitators set out to replicate the intervention used in the other cases with this important focus.

Several changes took place during this process that distinguished this experience from the previous projects. In this case, the classroom teacher also served as a facilitator which ensured that she would develop a vested interest in the project's success. In addition, a graduate student from a local university joined the project midyear to observe the process and serve as a classroom aide. The class size was smaller, with all 24 students choosing to participate. This smaller group enabled the facilitators to have a closer working relationship with individual students. During the culture circle and discussion sessions, more students were able to express their ideas about the topic.

In contrast with the two previous cases where the facilitators clearly defined the general subject for study, students participating in this project were able to choose the health topic that was most important to them. Thus, the level of participation here was broader than in the previous cases and more closely attuned to the Freirean problem-posing methodology. Students once again directed all phases of project development and were able to explore and give voice to the influence that violence was having on their lives and in their community.

Gangstar, One Shot At Life tells the story of a character's experience with gang involvement, the events that precipitated his choice to become involved with a gang, and the consequences of that decision. Other social issues such as child abuse, substance use and peer pressure were also featured as part of the storyline.

Students received recognition from many arenas for their work on the photonovel, and were extremely proud when the Mayor of Boston wrote to them and acknowledged their efforts in his Safe Neighborhoods Plan. In addition, the local newspaper highlighted their project in a feature story. A schoolwide celebration was held to distribute the newly published booklets and served to bring closure to the process. Students were enthusiastic participants. They too, wanted to use the photonovel as a teaching tool because they were concerned about the effect gangs were having on younger students. Although time constraints prohibited the peer teaching component from becoming fully developed, the facilitators were able to take the completed booklets to other schools and use them to spur discussions about the health topic.

Evaluation results yielded positive findings. There were some unexpected consequences as well. While gang violence was perceived by the majority of students as a major threat to health, some students also wanted to address additional topics. They requested a forum where they could talk openly about subjects such as HIV/AIDS, teen pregnancy and relationships. The facilitators responded to this request by proposing a once-a-week session where the group could come together to discuss these issues over lunch. Each week two students served as co-chairs of this lunch-time meeting and selected a topic for an informal presentation. "Brown Bag Lunch" continued throughout the year and became an important educational tool and vehicle of support for the students.

The articulation of a need and the active participation of students in a support group structured by them demonstrated to the facilitators that signs of empowerment were already being practiced. Students wanted more of a voice than was being offered through the materials production process. Through this dialogue, facilitators were able to problem pose with the students regarding various issues and helped them brainstorm possible solutions. This format allowed the facilitators to continue with their role as guides, thus strengthening and reinforcing the practice of collaborative learning that began with the photonovel.

Case 4: Peer Pressure

In the fourth materials production program, the facilitators wanted to further develop the process of collaborative learning and expand the peer teaching component. To ensure adequate time to accomplish these goals, this project was initiated with seventh-grade students and continued through the eighth grade. The first year resulted in the actual production of the booklet and the second year was devoted to the development of supplemental materials and peer teaching.

Students, as in the third case, were able to choose the topic that was most important to them as the theme of their project. *Friends: Are They Worth Dying For?* outlines the apprehension and anxiety students feel when they must start a new school and the temptation to try drugs as a way of gaining acceptance and coping in a new setting.

Because the production process was extended over a period of time, there were numerous opportunities for the school community to embrace and support the project. Faculty and staff participated in fundraising, provided assistance with assignments, and consented to portray the adult roles needed to complete the storyline depicted in the photonovel. In addition to public health nurse facilitators, a classroom parent volunteered to help with the project. This parent provided a valuable link with other classroom parents and was able to communicate informally with them about the project's progress. In addition, she shared with facilitators the enthusiasm about the project that students expressed to her outside of the classroom setting.

Overall, the process was similar to that in the first three cases with some minor differences. As the project began to unfold it became apparent that these seventh graders needed more time to develop group-related skills. The two-year timeline helped facilitators structure activities to meet this need. Throughout the two-year process, students remained committed to this project and it became an important component of their school experience. During the second year, the students' primary teacher became ill and subsequently died. Students, determined to do something very special in her memory, decided to dedicate the photonovel to her.

As with previous efforts, students involved in this project developed a teachers' guide. However, unlike the previous cases, students were also able to use these materials to conduct classes about their topic of peer pressure and substance use for the younger students in grades five and six. In addition, they created student worksheets, such as word searches and crossword puzzles, to help augment key concepts that were identified in their book. Students took pride in their product and the younger recipients enjoyed both the materials and the lessons.

Reflections

There are several key components responsible for the successful implementation of these materials development programs. Facilitation is a critical aspect of a successful process. Attention to student needs and the development of group-related skills are both important ingredients and must be built into program design. In addition, practitioners must attend to organizational issues and garner institutional support before program implementation.

The Role of the Facilitator

The facilitator's role throughout the preceding projects was to introduce and guide students through the collaborative learning process with the goal of encouraging them to take a more active role in their education. Overall, a facilitator focuses on the process—establishing and maintaining an atmosphere conducive to sharing and collaboration, encouraging the active participation of all members of the working group. In each case, the facilitators provided a forum for the students to explore their feelings openly and express their concerns about health issues that were important to them. The supportive environment enabled students to express their needs, identify issues and problems in their lives, and strategize about potential solutions. Throughout this process the facilitator listened to and encouraged group discussion regarding the health topic while also serving as a resource person for the students. The facilitator may support the group, clarify options and provide technical assistance when needed. Freire would consider this role of the educator as a catalyst who facilitates group process to help uncover group values and underlying assumptions (Miner and Ward, 1992).

It is important to recognize that one is working with a powerful learning tool and that such a project might elicit a wide range of behaviors from both participants and observers. Thus, facilitators may need to serve as the liaison between the working group and the program sponsors or institution and may need to delineate boundaries and offer needed referrals. Furthermore, the facilitators need to serve as role models for both students and teachers, demonstrating for them the richness of the collaborative learning experience. For this reason, a minimum of two facilitators is highly recommended. This provides an opportunity for reflection and analysis. Regularly scheduled post-meeting discussions prove insightful and quite useful for planning the next session. For the three urban cases, the facilitators were able to enhance their skills and renew their commitment to the empowerment theory of education as they progressed along with the students and most certainly with each subsequent project.

Growth and Needed Skills

Empowerment education and the participatory learning process were new to many of the students who took part in these programs. Abilities needed, such as organizational and negotiating skills and the capability to problem solve, were often lacking.

Assessing the students' strengths at the beginning of the program allowed the facilitators to modify the process to encourage growth and to meet the students' needs. Opening exercises, such as conducting a force field analysis and engaging in values clarification exercises, were designed to provide easy entry into the process and also introduce new skills and build on existing ones. Over time, students grew accustomed to discussion sessions, became familiar with a less directive facilitators' role, and learned how to relate to adults in new ways.

Some students, uncomfortable at first with their new freedoms and responsibilities, were unable to control their behaviors and "acted out" during the process. This became one of the greatest challenges of the project—allowing students the latitude to create their photonovel while providing a structure in which they could work and grow. To accomplish this, individual students were asked to meet with the facilitators after school to discuss their behaviors during the class. After identifying the unacceptable behaviors and taking responsibility for them, students were asked to sit out the next session and reflect on what had happened. They were questioned as to whether they were committed to returning to the project. Many students had difficulty at first articulating what they had done, and, more important, why they might have acted in a disruptive manner. Alternative assignments were available for students who did not want to participate; however, all students chose to return to the project and only one student needed to meet with the facilitators twice.

For many students, the sensitive nature of the topic chosen for the program was anxiety producing. Often the problems being discussed were directly affecting their personal lives, and the "storyline" was too close to their reality for comfort. This was true for all four cases. The use of drugs and tobacco, drinking and driving, and violence were all issues with which students had firsthand experience. Facilitators must recognize this possibility and help these students navigate through the process. Acknowledging, at the start of the project, that grappling with these issues is not easy, allowing students to distance themselves when they feel it is necessary, and offering individual counseling are all ways to assist students who are having difficulty during the process. Having more than one facilitator in the classroom allows those not actively teaching to assess the students and intervene as needed.

Institutional Support

In order for programs such as these to succeed, institutional support is a critical factor. Project staff must negotiate the proposed intervention with the appropriate school administrative personnel. Prior to negotiation, it is helpful to frame the process by applying a systems theory method of analysis in order to assess and correct for potential failure points in the project's design. Figure 3 offers an illustration of a checklist for addressing issues of institutional support. This discussion draws from Orlandi et al. (1990) who suggest a careful examination and assessment of the diffusion process.

Success may be limited if the project fails to bring about its intended effect. This can occur if a project, though highly touted, has been poorly designed, inadequately evaluated or dishonestly represented. Therefore, it is vital that the goals and objectives of the program be clearly communicated to the administrators. Evaluation results of similar programs should be shared at this time. By doing so, there can be no misunderstanding regarding what the project has been designed to accomplish.

Ongoing, effective communication among all program participants must be a priority. A program can be genuinely efficacious and have the potential to achieve its intended effect yet fail to do so because it was communicated ineffectively. As the facilitators

Figure 3
Evaluation Checklist for the Successful
Diffusion of Programs in the School Setting

System Analysis	Yes	No	Changes

1. Does the program's design reflect its intended effect? Have goals, objectives and past evaluations been shared with the administrative staff?

2. Have the program goals, objectives and process been communicated to all members of the school community? faculty, staff, parents, community leaders, program participants, media?

3. Are there conflicts between the organization's values and beliefs and those introduced in the program?

4. Are there adequate resources to ensure completion of the project? funds, equipment, space, time?

5. Do any of the project components need to be eliminated? Are these vital to the project's success?

6. Are there mechanisms in place to ensure that the project's momentum is sustained over time?

evaluated each project it became clear that continuing communication was necessary on all levels. Administrative and support staff along with faculty, parents, community leaders, media and program participants needed to be kept apprised about the project's progress. Weekly written updates on the project's development helped keep everyone informed, involved and vested on some level with the project's outcome.

Success of the project will be in jeopardy if there is an incompatibility between program and organizational values and beliefs. The facilitators should be familiar with the sponsoring institution's philosophy and be prepared to make adjustments to the project if necessary.

Programs can also fail if there is a lack of necessary resources and allotted time. These resources and time commitments need to be identified at the beginning of the project and negotiated with the administrative staff. The materials production process must have, at minimum:

- adequate space for meetings and committee work
- access to simple props and space to photograph scenes for the booklet
- use of a typewriter or computer to help with dialogue development
- use of a camera

Printing facilities and costs must be established and planned for at the program start. Furthermore, the project requires a degree of flexibility with students' schedules for time-consuming activities such as photography sessions.

Some interventions are not implemented because specific program components (such as instructor training) which are considered instrumental to the program's efficacy are omitted or drastically abbreviated. Facilitators must clearly delineate those elements of the process that cannot be eliminated without compromising the success of the project (Orlandi et al., 1990). In one of the cases described, administrators questioned the need for a culture circle—believing that such a forum could result in increased noise and confusion. The facilitators acknowledged that while the booklet could be produced without this activity, they felt it was vital to the process for students to discuss the health problem they had chosen in a forum such as this. When the rationale for and the importance of the culture circle were explained, it remained part of the project.

As is the case with many projects, the process and focus can begin to lose momentum and dissipate rapidly over time. Establishing mechanisms to ensure that the spirit of the program is sustained over time is one of the great challenges for the facilitator. Students, while initially excited about a new learning opportunity, need periodic reinforcement that what they are doing is important and valued. During these materials development projects, that reinforcement came from positive letters home to parents, feedback from community leaders or media, and frequent inquiries about the process from faculty and support staff to the students. In addition, fundraisers that promoted enjoyable activities such as making and selling Valentine's Day cards or putting on a talent show to raise money for the booklet helped generate a spirit of cooperation and enthusiasm.

Participatory materials development programs can be successfully implemented within school settings if careful attention is given to the methodology associated with diffusing these innovations (Orlandi et al., 1990). By examining the program for potential failure points prior to negotiation with administrative staff, flaws in the organization, design, adoption and delivery can be identified and adjusted to ensure a greater chance of success.

Conclusion

Empowerment education programs are wonderful vehicles for learning. As students focus on communicating important information to others, they have an opportunity to be more reflective about what they want to say, how they want to say it, and why it is important for others to pay attention. Participatory materials development provides a vehicle for students to be creative, to manage a project, and to be in control. Most important, perhaps, is the added benefit of enabling students to reflect on their own experiences and use those experiences as the foundation for additional learning. There are benefits for the product as well. Materials developed by students for other students tap into the shared culture, ground the topics at hand in the reality of students' lives, and give voice to the idiom of current speech.

Often health educators will come to students with predefined parameters of a contract or grant and with the focus or health concern already articulated. As long as the limits are clearly defined and students still have the opportunities to introduce issues of importance to them, the participatory project can go well. As is evident in the first case, students can bring creativity and energy to topics not in their first priority listing. The programs are stronger, however, when students are able to determine and focus on areas of major concern to them. The latter cases under discussion offer strong examples of serious determination among a group of students to address key issues of importance to their daily lives. In one of the cases, simply focusing on a topic of interest to the students served to open doors to further discussion.

Today's students grapple with profoundly disturbing threats to their health and well-being. They need information and skills, opportunities to explore issues and seek solutions, a chance to collaborate with peers and supportive adults. Community- and school-based health education efforts can make an important contribution to their lives through programs that attend to process as well as content and that are designed to become vehicles for empowerment. Participatory materials development can be one aspect of such a comprehensive effort.

We offer our thanks and appreciation to John P. Comings, EdD, Daniel M. Merrigan, SJ, EdD, Lillian Shirley, RN, MPH, Karen Hacker, MD, and Dorothy MacKenzie, RN.

References

Allensworth, D., and L. Kolbe. 1987. The comprehensive school health program: Exploring an expanded concept. *Journal of School Health* 57 (10): 409-412.

Bandura, A. 1986. *Social Foundations of Thought and Action: A Social Cognitive Theory.* Englewood Cliffs, NJ: Prentice-Hall.

Brown, C. 1974. Literacy in 30 hours: Paulo Freire's process in Northeast Brazil. *Social Policy* 5 (2): 25-32.

CASPAR Alcohol Education Program. 1987. *Decisions about drinking: A sequential alcohol education curriculum.* Somerville, MA.

Center for International Education. 1975. *Non-formal education in Ecuador 1971-1975.* Amherst, MA: University of Massachusetts.

Comings, J. P. 1979. The participatory development of materials and media for nonformal education. Dissertation. Amherst: University of Massachusetts.

Comings, J. P., S. C. Franz and B. C. Cain. 1981. Community participation in environmental health education materials. *Convergence* 14 (2): 36-44.

Flay, B. 1985. Psychosocial approaches to smoking prevention: A review of the findings. *Health Psychology* 5 (April): 451.

Freire, P. 1968a. *Education for Critical Consciousness.* New York: The Seabury Press.

Freire, P. 1968b. *Pedagogy of the Oppressed.* New York: The Seabury Press.

McGinnis, J. M., and C. DeGraw. 1991. Healthy schools 2000: Creating partnerships for the decade. *Journal of School Health* 61 (7): 292-297.

Miner, K. J., and S. E. Ward. 1992. Ecological health promotion: The promise of empowerment education. *Journal of Health Promotion* 23 (7): 429-432.

Minkler, M., and K. Cox. 1980. Creating critical consciousness in health: Applications of Freire's philosophy and methods to the health care setting. *International Journal of Health Services* 10 (2): 311-322.

Orlandi, M. A., C. Landers, R. Weston and N. Haley. 1990. Diffusion of health promotion innovations. In *Health Behavior and Health Education*, ed. K. Glanz, F. M. Lewis and B. Rimer, 288-313. San Francisco, CA: Jossey-Bass.

Roter, D. L., R. E. Rudd, J. Keogh and B. Robinson. 1987. Worker produced health education material for the construction trades. *International Quarterly of Community Health Education* 7 (2): 109-121.

Rudd, R. E., and J. M. Kichen. 1980. Participatory health education materials development. Presentation to the American Public Health Association Annual Meeting, Detroit, Michigan, October.

Rudd, R. E., J. M. Kichen and I. Joslin. 1980. *Student produced health education material: A "how-to" manual.* Easthampton, MA: Lifeways.

Shorr, I. 1987. *Freire for the classroom: A sourcebook for liberatory teaching.* Portsmouth, NH: Boynton/Cook.

Wallerstein, N., and E. Bernstein. 1988. Empowerment education: Freire's ideas adapted to health education. *Health Education Quarterly* 15 (4): 379-394.

Chapter 10

Working Cooperatively with Native-American Communities to Educate Children and Youth

Michael E. Bird, MSW, MPH,
William M. Kane, PhD, CHES,
Lisa Shames, PhD, and Mark Jager, MS

The children of Indian Tribes which have kept close touch with the world of nature and with their indigenous cultures are specially stimulated to observe accurately, to organize accurately their observations and express them aesthetically...White children and urban White children especially, may have much less chance to form concepts from firsthand observation, but must rely more upon books and words (Havinghurst, Gunther and Pratt, 1946).

Prior to "the discovery of America" by Columbus there were an estimated 2.5 million indigenous people representing 300 distinct tribal cultures living in what now constitutes the United States. That number had dwindled to an estimated 250,000 by the late 1800s. Disease, warfare/extermination and government-sponsored relocation were all factors which contributed to the death of more than 90 percent of these societies. American Indians have demonstrated amazing durability and persistence in human survival when faced with onslaught from other cultures. America's educational system has been one of the partners in this onslaught.

Today, approximately 1.5 million American Indians and Alaska Natives representing 512 federally recognized Tribes reside in the United States. In general there is much in common that these populations share. The first self-identifier for Indian people is usually membership in or affiliation with a specific tribe or tribes. More than 50 percent are under fifty years of age. Approximately 50 percent live on the Reservation or in the Pueblo, and 50 percent live away from their traditional home. There is much movement between the traditional home and urban areas. The average educational level of adults is ninth grade. Between 80 and 95 percent of those who enter college leave before the end of the first year. Unemployment among American Indians ranges from 50 to 80 percent. The average annual income is less than $2,000. Eighty percent of the women earn an annual salary of less than $4,000.

For purposes of clarity in this chapter it is necessary to define several terms which we will use in our discussion of Native People of America. The term "Native People" will be used to describe all people of the now United States whose ancestral occupation of this land predates Columbus' "discovery of America" in 1492. Native People include 323 "American Indian" Tribes officially recognized by the federal government; more than 500 "Alaska Natives" and "Eskimo" groups; and indigenous "Pacific Islanders" of the Hawaiian Islands. This chapter will focus on American Indians—their culture, family values and social political environments, which have implications for teachers and health educators working in schools.

American Indian Belief Systems: Implications for Health Education

Despite the commonalities among Tribes, each Tribe has its own historical, social, cultural, political and economic uniqueness. More than 300 languages are spoken by these Native Peoples. Geographically these Tribes are dispersed throughout the United States with each group making the necessary adaptions unique to their environs. Traditional values, religious practices and family structures differ greatly, with each Tribe having its own unique set of beliefs. Although each Tribe is unique, Locust (1985) has described the following as a more or less common set of health beliefs. This set of health beliefs is provided as a guide for health educators and is not meant to be universally ascribed to all Indian communities.

- There is a Supreme Creator, and there are also lesser beings.
- Each human is multidimensional being made up of a body, a mind and a spirit.
- Plants and animals, like humans, are part of the spirit world. This spirit world coexists and intermingles with the physical world.
- The spirit existed before it came into a physical body and will exist after the body dies.
- Illness affects the mind and spirit as well as the body.
- Wellness is harmony in body, mind and spirit.
- Unwellness is disharmony in body, mind and spirit.
- Natural unwellness is caused by violation of a sacred or tribal taboo.
- Unnatural unwellness is caused by witchcraft.
- Individuals are responsible for their own wellness.

Beck and Walters (1977) have identified other beliefs which have implications for teachers and health educators working with American Indian children and youth. Again, it is necessary to caution that belief can differ greatly from Tribe to Tribe. The following beliefs help provide some understanding of the American Indian's view of relationships among individuals, families, communities, Tribes, peoples of the world, the cosmos and the Creator.

- There are unseen powers, or what some people call the Great Mystery or Great Spirit.
- All things in the universe are dependent on each other. American Indians see themselves as part of the environment, not masters with a need to control the environment.
- Personal worship reinforces the bonds between the individual, the community and the great powers. Worship is a personal commitment to the sources of life.
- Sacred traditions and persons knowledgeable in them are responsible for teaching morals and ethics.
- Most communities and Tribes have trained practitioners who have been given names such as Medicine Man, Priest, Shaman and Cacique. These individuals, who may also have titles specific to each Tribe, are responsible for specialized, perhaps secret knowledge. They help pass knowledge and sacred practices from generation to generation, storing what they know in their memories.
- Humor is a necessary part of the sacred. Human beings are often weak—we are not gods—and our weakness leads us to do foolish things; therefore, clowns and similar figures are needed to show us how we act and why.

It is difficult to contrast the value systems of American Indians with those of Whites. American Indians, like Whites, have many value systems. Keeping this in mind, American Indians in general place the importance of the group above the value of the individual. Other commonly shared values include respect for elders; importance of sharing with family and community; orientation to present time; allegiance to family, friends and community; and living in harmony with nature. From a social and public health point of view, these values hold great potential and represent strengths upon which health educators can build when working with Indian children, youth and families.

Culturally Specific Health Education

An ultimate goal of health education is that it be both culturally specific and multicultural. Culturally specific education for American Indian children and youth requires that those delivering the education have full understanding of and respect for the historical, traditional and cultural values of the specific Tribe, community and family. In order for health education programs to be culturally specific, they must be developed in concert with the child's family and community, and respect and enhance the values of that population. In this process, the health educator becomes a consultant to the community in development of appropriate programs.

Health educators as consultants need more than knowledge of school-based programs, health issues, teaching and learning strategies, curriculum development, and implementation and evaluation expertise. Health educators need to:

- Understand the historical, traditional and cultural values unique to the Tribe, community and family.
- Develop skills which enable them to engage community members and leaders in efforts to define their future aspirations for their children and youth.

- Work with community leaders to interpret health education theories and principles that serve as the basis for curriculum development.
- Work with community leaders in the development of culturally appropriate curricula, learning and teaching strategies, and classroom materials.
- Promote health education, training and employment opportunities for Indian people who because of their commitment are most likely to remain in the community.
- Identify community leaders, elders and family members who can be involved in working with teachers to deliver instruction for children and youth and provide classroom learning experiences based on the specific culture, tradition, values and learning styles of the community.
- Work with community leaders to help family members acquire the skills which support health education being delivered through the schools.

Many American Indians, especially elders and those who are in close touch with the traditional cultures of the Tribes, place high value on honesty, trust, integrity and sincerity. Many have an uncanny ability to sense integrity and sincerity in others. An elder once described the development of the sense as akin to development of other senses (smell, taste, hearing). He described it as a sense that his people have honed to a fine art as a result of generations of interacting with outsiders, many of whom were interested in personal gains and not the good of the Tribe. Honesty, integrity and sincerity are not skills that can be developed by health educators. They are innate qualities. Health educators who are not honest, accepting and sincere will not trusted (nor should they be) by tribal leaders to develop and deliver health education programs to Indian children and youth.

Multicultural Health Education

Multicultural health education is more than education about the health issues and concerns of multiple cultures. Multicultural education builds on the strengths of various cultures, enabling children and youth of all cultures to acquire knowledge, wisdom and an appreciation for the needs, hopes and dreams of other cultures.

Multicultural education enhances the potential for all children of the world to be able to develop more than one set of lenses for viewing life. Appreciating differences and recognizing the strengths of diverse cultures and community and family values is a critical component of multicultural health education. Many children and youth (and adults) live in a monoculture (e.g., only rural, poor Hispanic; upper-middle-class White; or poor, southern African American). These children imagine that everyone and everywhere is just like them and their immediate community.

Children who grow up experiencing and valuing only their own culture are culturally disadvantaged. They are able to view other cultures only through their own cultural lens. Therefore, these children (and adults) often find behaviors and customs of other cultures bizarre, amusing or romantic. These culturally disadvantaged children become adults (and some teachers) who are unable to appreciate the strengths of diversity, and unable (and often unwilling) to accept diverse approaches to problem solving. They often have a need (and, unfortunately, the resources and power) to shape society to fit their own cultural values. The ultimate goal of a multicultural school health education program is to foster the development of children and youth who can utilize the strengths of many cultures as a foundation for developing healthy behaviors and lifestyles. American Indian cultures have much to offer all people interested in establishing healthy lifestyles.

Education of Indian Children and Youth

The history of formal education of Indian children and youth in this country is full of examples of mistakes made by the "dominant" society that attempted to control the educational process. The United States Government operates the Bureau of Indian Affairs (BIA), which has had primary responsibility for the formal education of Indian children and youth. A common past practice of the BIA was to remove children from their families and communities at an early age and ship them away to boarding school. Once at the boarding school and removed from their culture, their hair was cut, they were taught English and often punished for speaking their native tongue, their traditional clothes were discarded and they were put into western clothes and uniforms, and practice of all traditional beliefs was discouraged (often with punishment). They were reinforced for their acceptance (and often punished for refusal) of Anglo culture and values, the English language and foreign learning styles.

Ortiz (1972) summarized his perception of the problem of Indian education: "At the very least we may assume that while the [Indian] parents do their job, the schools do not; indeed, the schools actually negate the parents' initial success in presenting a normal, well-adjusted six-year-old to the school."

Cahn (1969) asserted that Indian people learned three lessons from the BIA:

1. Indian people's attempts at self-realization are almost always frustrated. The BIA denies the Indians, individually and as a group, the right to make decisions that affect their immediate lives. The results are feelings of powerlessness and frustration and acceptance of the futility of planning for the future.
2. Dependency is a virtue.

3. Alienation is rewarded. Indians who reject their language, birthplace, people and culture in favor of White culture are rewarded with economic security.

Unfortunately, the only alternatives in the past to the BIA schools were the missionary schools operated by organized religions. Many of these schools also spent great amounts of energy attempting to convert children from their native spiritual beliefs and practices to Christianity. This often was accompanied by efforts to get children to reject their culture, traditions and "heathen" pasts. Indian children's success in these schools was dependent upon rejecting the strengths of their family and community values and culture and accepting the Anglo culture. The suspicion and distrust of White educators that many American Indians harbor are accurate perceptions based on almost 500 years of history.

Little Soldier (1992) identified five value differences that often cause discontinuity between children, school and home. A teacher's awareness of these value differences is a first step in understanding American Indian children and youth in the classroom.

1. Direct personal criticism and harsh discipline that might negatively influence a child's self-esteem are avoided in the home.
2. Native American children may feel indifference to acquiring material goods.
3. Many Native Americans tend to view time as flowing and relative; things are done as the need arises rather than by the clock or according to some future-oriented master plan.
4. Not all children, and certainly not all Native American children, learn best in the logical, linear and sequential teaching style typical of today's schools.
5. Physical modesty should be considered; the need for privacy in toileting, dressing/undressing, and showering in physical education classes must be taken into account.

Today, many young Indian children attended local community schools operated by Tribal authorities. In the past, the sparse populations of most reservations and pueblos often meant children were transported long distances and frequently attended non-Tribal-operated high schools. This too is slowly changing, with more Tribes operating their own high schools. In addition, Indian parents are becoming more involved in the education of their children when they attend schools off the Reservation or Pueblo.

Learning Styles: Implication for Classroom Teachers

American Indian children and youth not only have unique cultures but have learning styles and strengths unique to their cultures. In addition, Indian families have unique teaching styles.

Until recently, learning styles have not been a major interest of teachers. Schools and teachers charged with the responsibility of educating children and youth have traditionally focused on the content which society has deemed important to master. Those who mastered the content were rewarded with praise, good grades and future opportunities. Those who did not master the content were ignored or labeled as "slow learners" or, in today's jargon, "children at risk." Many, perhaps most, American Indian children fell into these categories. A major reason for this was that the learning styles and strengths of American Indian children were not acknowledged by teachers, and the teaching styles of these teachers were inconsistent with the needs of Indian children.

But not all schools serving Indian children and youth were bad. Johns-Steiner (1975) described Pueblo classrooms where children's culture and individual approaches to learning were reinforced and yet these students assimilated both "academic" content and process. Unfortunately, many schools do not recognize or affirm these strengths. The devaluation, whether intentional, or unintentional due to ignorance, of the strengths of Indian children profoundly affects these children's classroom performance. Teachers and schools that do not value the strengths of the child's culture precipitate a rift between the family and community and the school.

Several scholars have described the overnight change which occurs among bright, vibrant Indian children who move from a local Indian-community-operated school, where the teacher and classroom support and extend culturally familiar learning styles, to a school in an outside community where cultural support is lacking, native language usage and development is discouraged and learning styles are foreign (Johns-Steiner, 1975; Little Soldier, 1992; Ortiz, 1972). These children soon become sullen, silent and low achievers.

Identification of learning styles of students and structuring of learning activities to build on the strengths of each individual's learning style has received more attention by health educators in recent years. The following are characteristics of learning styles identified among some American Indian populations.

Learning through Observation and Practice
Indian children learn by observing and listening in their homes and communities. Indian parents supplement their modeling of behavior with an emphasis on verbal rules and explanations when interacting with their children. These parents take seriously the necessity of children understanding the reasons for an event or activity. Johns-Steiner (1975) reports the opportunity for Pueblo Indian children to observe their elders at work, over long stretches of time, as one aspect which was significantly related to cognitive development. She hypothesized that one reason that observational learning was significant was that such learning takes place

among people with whom the child is emotionally involved. She suggests that effective observational learning involves large sequences of activity with a continuum of involvement. American Indian children learn by first observing; and then taking a progressively larger and larger role in the performance of activities as they grow older.

Learning from Storytelling

Parents and elder community members teach by demonstration and storytelling. Interviews with Pueblo adults found that they always tied their descriptions of learning experiences to adult family members. Their most significant models were described as people one or two generations older than themselves. Tribal traditions, history and community social norms are often communicated and passed down from generation to generation through these stories. Exposure of Indian children to learning activities and processes which lack complexity and continuity are of little use for significant kinds of learning (Johns-Steiner, 1975).

Learning Metaphorically

Symbolism, anthropomorphism (giving human characteristics to animals, gods and objects), animism (giving life and soul to natural phenomena such as rocks, trees and wind) and metaphors are techniques which seem to enable Indian children to master complex concepts (More, 1987). Havinghurst, Gunther and Pratt (1946) described Indian children who have kept in close touch with the world of nature and with their culture as more able to observe accurately, organize their observations and express them aesthetically than White children who have less chance to form concepts from firsthand observation and rely more on books and words.

Learning by Trial and Error

Independent thinking and action are valued, and trial and error is often an important and honored learning process in American Indian homes and communities. Parents do not expect their children to perform in a short time and American Indian families seldom rebuke their children for making mistakes (Johns-Steiner, 1975; Little Soldier, 1992).

Learning Through Play

At an early age, Indian children are provided the opportunity to learn through play and exploration. Dramatic presentations and expression through artwork are extensions of the learning through play concept at which many American Indian children excel.

Learning Cooperatively

The cultural emphasis placed on the importance of the group as opposed to the individual results in Indian children who have no pressure to perform individually and "stand out" (Swisher and Deyhle, 1989). In fact, many Indian children consider it inappropriate behavior to rise to the teacher's challenge to perform individually in class.

As a result, many Indian children have no urge or motivation to outdo other students in the classroom. Indian students prefer cooperative group learning and projects over small- or large-group recitation.

Teacher-organized competition between students is not a motivating factor for many Indian students. Teachers who use stars to reward outstanding work may actually be discouraging performance (Gilliland, 1988). Because many Indian students are not motivated by competition or because they refuse to become active participants in recitation, they may be perceived and labeled as dull or uninterested.

Learning Through Reflection

The Indian learner prefers a reflective approach to a task. Students show respect to the teacher and the task through quiet, thoughtful introspection. Often students will feel no need to volunteer answers and they may respond only after careful reflection. A typical teacher who demands immediate responses from students will not evoke a response from many Indian students.

Learning as a Private Experience

American Indian children often learn under the guidance of trusted elders as a private affair in many Indian societies. Likewise testing and correcting are also conducted in private. The emphasis in Indian communities is on learning. On the other hand, "teaching" is de-emphasized in an attempt to allow Indian children to develop their own observational abilities and insight. The Indian learner is encouraged to "self-test" in privacy before attempting a task. A sign of respect to the task is performance with a minimum of error. Public testing, and especially the standardized testing conducted in most schools today, is in direct opposition to the values and learning styles of most Indian children.

Designing and Delivering Multicultural School Health Education

The challenge for those responsible for developing and delivering multicultural school-based health education programs is to meld the theory and science of health education and health behavior with the strengths of all cultures to produce programs which benefit all children. The development of programs which build on the specific cultural strengths of American Indian populations is a first priority for those working with Indian children and youth.

Building on the Concept of Globalness

School health educators designing programs for American Indian children and youth need to build on the strengths presented by Indians' understanding of the concept of globalness. The ability of Indian children to conceptualize total systems should be reflected in health education programs designed to meet their needs. The relationships between theory and science, curriculum and program components, and learning activities need to be evident to the students and their families. Whole concepts or snapshot pictures of the whole should be presented to students prior to breaking skills into isolated small segments.

Health educators recognize that knowledge plays only a small role in students' development of healthy behaviors. Teachers should clearly identify the relationship between essential knowledge and the skills and experiences children and youth need to practice healthy behaviors. Kane (1993) has proposed that children need a combination of health knowledge and skills and must be presented with the opportunity to practice these healthy skills in the school, home and community. Reinforcement that children and youth receive when these healthy skills are demonstrated plays a major role in the future practice of these healthy behaviors. Children who receive either internal satisfaction, external praise, rewards or benefits, are more likely to continue the healthy behaviors. The ability of Indian children to reward themselves and the supportive roles the parents and elders of these children play are strengths which will tend to support the continued practice of healthy behaviors.

The expectations and values of each individual and the social norms of the family, peers, the community and the schools are important factors in determining the reinforcement children and youth receive for the practice of healthy behaviors. Establishing the interconnectiveness of health knowledge, skills, opportunities to practice, and reinforcement from the classroom, peers, family members and community is a starting point for school-based health educators working with American Indian children and youth.

Utilizing the Total Person Concept

Framing health education within the context of the total person, as proposed by Papenfuss (1994), is a second recommendation for those working with Indian children and youth. From birth, most Indian children have been raised to appreciate the importance of keeping the whole person healthy. Health education which builds on the relationship of body, mind and spirit is consistent with the cultural values of these children.

Risk-reduction concepts should incorporate opportunities for Indian children and youth to exercise their ability to see the whole versus the parts. Although development of specific resistance skills is essential, the opportunities for application of these skills through roleplaying and use of creative drama should increase the likelihood that these students will establish ongoing healthy behaviors.

Roleplaying as a Learning Strategy

Okwumabua and Duryea (1989) found that roleplay simulations and question/answer panel discussion sessions were successful in generating Indian student participation, communication and understanding of health decision making. These authors also report that health education teachers can build on the nonverbal communication skills of American Indian students to help them develop resistance skills. This is consistent with recommendations of others which suggest that classroom-based skills development should focus on observation over a long period of time followed by practice of the process, with a minimum of verbal interchange.

Establishing Peer Teaching Programs

The use of peer tutoring and cross-age teaching involving Indian children and youth and the use of family members and elders as lay educators in the classroom is an approach which is consistent with the learning styles of most Tribes. The opportunity for one student to exercise responsibility in helping other students has been shown to produce beneficial results in the area of health behaviors (Resnik and Gibbs, 1986). A typical pattern of learning in Indian communities is that of a younger person observing and learning from the examples and actions of older persons. The inclusion of family members and elders who act as lay educators provides continuity between community and school life. Elders are an extremely powerful role models for Indian children and youth.

Promoting Introspection in Health Decision Making

Thoughtful introspection of issues prior to responding is another cultural value of American Indians which might be embraced by health educators to enhance the education of all children. Health decision making requires introspection. The typical pattern of teacher questioning and students immediately responding has not served health educators interested in developing students' decision-making skills. Introspection is not something that will benefit just Indian children. Introspection prior to health decision making and action is a concept which should be borrowed from the Indian culture and become a foundation for all students.

Utilizing Visualization as a Learning Strategy

Teaching and learning techniques which allow American Indian children and youth to apply their finely developed skills in processing visual and spatial information should be routinely utilized. For example, the use of instructional games and play as learning and teaching techniques allows students to learn in a manner that utilizes their experiences. New health concepts and material should be presented in a visual or spatial modality rather than verbally. Ideas should be described in terms of metaphors, images, analogies and symbols rather than with dictionary definitions.

Cooperative Learning

Health education teachers need to strive continually to shift from efforts of the past 100 years that focused on teacher-directed learning to efforts that focus on student-directed learning. For more than two decades, school health educators have engaged students in cooperative learning. Continuing to explore cooperative learning strategies is an excellent example of building on the strengths of the American Indian cultures to enhance the development of all children and youth. Cooperative learning groups, a technique particularly appropriate for health education, should be utilized instead of traditional groupings by achievement or individual assignment, which have a tendency to foster competition.

Learning from American Indian Authors

Charles (1989) suggested that teachers should seek to include learning materials which contain representation of selections by American Indian authors from various regions of the United States. Many of the writings of American Indian authors are particularly relevant to the development of self-concept and make the connection between healthy physical, social, emotional, mental and spiritual aspects of human development. If Indian children and youth are going to develop to their optimal potential, development built upon the culture of these children is essential.

Granting Independence for Learners

The combination of the above experiences and upbringing results in American Indian children's development of self-confidence and independence at a very early age. This confidence, independence and vitality is often exhibited by young children in the classroom in schools where these strengths are recognized and affirmed. The ability to resist peer pressure to engage in risky health behaviors is enhanced by an individual's independence. Health educators should grant the necessary independence to students which enables them to continue to be independent learners.

Allowing Flexibility of Structure

Classroom structure that is informal and allows for freedom of movement (small informal groups or circles, sitting at tables) provides a more conducive learning environment for most Indian children and youth. Rigid classroom structures and environment tend to force Indian children to withdraw. Opportunities which enable children to practice healthy skills require a maximum of structural and scheduling flexibility.

The Health Educator as an Advocate for Learning

Health educators have an ethical responsibility to serve as advocates for all children and youth. Schools especially need professional advocates who understand the unique needs of poor and ethnically diverse populations. Without effective advocates who can bring about change, schools have a tendency to continue to operate as they have operated in the past. Past educational practices have done little to meet the needs of American Indian children and youth.

Greenburg (1992) suggests that teachers interested in embracing a multicultural and anti-bias classroom curriculum speak up about their own lack of knowledge and appropriate materials and uncertainties as to what to do and how to deliver culturally specific education. She suggests that teachers should ask the school to:

- Establish regular interaction with American Indian resource people.
- Establish ongoing collaboration with local, state or national American Indians who specialize in educating people about aspects of American Indians' lives and issues today as well as issues in the past.
- Adapt existing resources and create new materials that enable the inclusion of authentic yet developmentally appropriate information into the existing curriculum.
- Establish inservice training conducted by American Indian individuals and organizations.

Programs Serving American Indian Children and Youth

There is a growing number of materials and programs designed for American Indian children and youth of which health education specialists should be aware. The following is a brief description of some of these materials and programs. Complete addresses and telephone numbers for each project can be found at the end of this chapter.

Three Feathers Associates has developed several projects including a health curriculum for children "Growing Up Strong." In addition, the organization has developed a resource center, which includes health education materials, for Head Start directors.

United National Indian Tribal Youth (UNITY) has developed material designed to provide leadership opportunities for Indian Youth. These include goals for Indian Youth for the Year 2000.

Northwest Indian Child Welfare Institute has developed a variety of materials and programs for prevention of child abuse and developing positive child-rearing skills based on Indian traditions.

American Indian Health Care Association has funding from the U.S. Office of Disease Prevention and Health Promotion to assist with the development of programs and materials to facilitate the achievement of Year 2000 Health Objectives.

Adolescent Initiative developed by the American Medical Association is a monograph which includes guidance for health care providers in their work with American Indian adolescents.

Bilingual Education Multifunctional Resource Center located at the University of Oklahoma produces a wide range of materials on tradition, health beliefs and learning styles of American Indian children and youth.

After School Care Program, a Cooperative Extension Service funded project at Muskogee, Oklahoma, has developed a wide range of health education materials and learning activities for the development of self-concept and health behaviors based on tradition and culture.

Four Worlds Development Project, out of the Faculty of Education at the University of Lethbridge, Alberta, Canada, has developed materials for teachers who are working with Native children and youth.

Albuquerque Area Indian Health Service and the State of New Mexico, in conjunction with the IHS, have developed a school health curriculum (Ristra) to meet the needs of New Mexico's diverse population. New Mexico's population includes 19 Pueblo Tribes, two Apache Tribes and two Navajo Tribes. The Ristra curriculum was developed utilizing input from these populations.

Pathways to Health, developed at the University of New Mexico, is a program that focuses on prevention of cardiovascular disease and cancer through curriculum development at the elementary school level.

National Native American AIDS Prevention Center has developed a wide range of educational materials designed to be utilized with American Indian populations. These include materials targeting drug and alcohol misuse, and indiscriminate sexual behaviors.

Resources

Administration for Native
   Americans
200 Independence Ave. SW
Washington, DC 20201
Attention: CDP 90-1
(202) 245-7727

Americans for Indian Opportunity
3508 Garfield St. NW
Washington, DC 20007
(202) 338-8809

American Indian and Alaska Native
   Caucus
American Public Health
   Association
1015 15th St. NW, Suite 300
Washington, DC 20005
(202) 789-5600

American Indian Health Care
   Association
245 East 6th St., Suite 499
St. Paul, MN 55101
(612) 293-0233

American Indian Institute
555 E. Constitution St.
Norman, OK 73037
(405) 325-1446

American Medical Association
Adolescent Initiative
515 North State St.
Chicago, IL 60610
(312) 464-5000

Association of American Indian
   Physicians
10015 S. Pennsylvania
Oklahoma City, OK 73159
(405) 692-1202

Four Worlds Development Project
Faculty of Education
University of Lethbridge
4401 University Dr.
Lethbridge, Alberta, T1K3MA
Canada
(403) 328-4343

Indian Health Service
5600 Fishers Lane
Rockville, MD 20857
(301) 443-4297

National Association for Native
   American Children
   of Alcoholics
611 12 Ave. S, Suite 200
Seattle, WA 98144
(206) 324-9360

National American Indian AIDS
   Prevention Center
3515 Grand Ave., Suite 100
Oakland, CA 94616
(800) 283-2437

National Congress of American
   Indians
900 Pennsylvania Ave. SE
Washington, DC 20003
(202) 546-9404

National Indian Council on Aging
P. O. Box 2088
Albuquerque, NM 87103
(505) 242-9505

National Indian Health Board
50 S. Steele St., Suite 500
Denver, CO 80209
(303) 394-3500

Northwest Indian Child Welfare
Institute
P. O. Box 751
Portland, OR 97207
(503) 725-3038

Multicultural Substance Abuse
Prevention
Office of Substance Abuse
Prevention
P. O. Box 350A
Silver Spring, MD 20910
(800) 822-0047

Three Feathers Associates
P. O. Box 5508
Norman, OK 73070
(405) 360-2919

United National Indian Tribal
Youth, Inc.
P. O. Box 25042
Oklahoma City, OK 73125
(405) 423-3010

References

Beck, P. V, and A. L. Walters. 1977. *The sacred: Ways of knowledge, sources of life*. Tsaile, AZ: Navajo Community College Press.

Cahn, E., ed. 1969. *Our brother's keeper: The Indian in White America*. New York: New Community Press.

Charles, J. P. 1989. The need for textbook reform: An American Indian example. *Journal of American Indian Education* 28 (3): 24-27.

Gilliland, H. 1988. *Teaching the Native American*. Dubuque, IA: Kendal/Hunt.

Greenburg, P. 1992. Teaching about Native Americans? or teaching about people including Native Americans? *Young Children* (September): 27-30, 79-81.

Havinghurst, R. J., M. K. Gunther and I. E. Pratt. 1946. Environment and draw-a-man test: The performance of Indian children. *Journal of Abnormal and Social Psychology* 41:50-63.

Johns-Steiner, V. 1975. Learning styles among Pueblo children: Final report. Report to National Institute of Education, U.S. Department of Health, Education and Welfare, College of Education, University of New Mexico.

Kane, W. 1993. *Step by step to comprehensive school health: The program planning guide*. Santa Cruz, CA: ETR Associates.

Little Soldier, L. 1992. Working with Native American children. *Young Children* (September): 15-21.

Locust, C. 1985. *American Indian beliefs concerning health and unwellness.* Monograph Series of the Native American Research and Training Center. Tucson, AZ: University of Arizona.

More, A. J. 1987. Native Indian learning styles: A review for researchers and teachers. *Journal of American Indian Education* 26:17-29.

Okwumabua, J. O., and E. J. Duryea. 1989. A test of the ability of Native American seventh-grade students to learn and apply a four step decision making process. *Journal of American Indian Education* 28 (3): 14-23.

Ortiz A. 1972. Native education under fire. In *The American Indian Reader: Education,* 78-87. San Francisco, CA: The Indian Historian Press, Inc.

Papenfuss, R. L. 1994. Physical fitness: A vital component for total health and high-level wellness. In *The comprehensive school health challenge: Promoting health through education,* ed. P. Cortese and K. Middleton, 491-521. Santa Cruz, CA: ETR Associates.

Resnik H., and J. Gibbs. 1986. Types of peer program approaches. In *Adolescent peer pressure: Theory correlates, and program implications for drug abuse prevention,* 47-89. Rockville, MD: NIDA.

Swisher, K., and D. Deyhle. 1989. The styles of learning are different, but the teaching is just the same: Suggestions for teachers of American Indian youth. *Journal of American Indian Education* 28 (3): 28-32.

Chapter 11

Teaching Health Through Sheltered English

Lillian Vega Castaneda, EdD

This chapter provides an overview and explanation of specially designed academic instruction for English language learners. It focuses on "sheltered English" as an instructional approach in teaching health content.

The first section offers a definition of sheltered instruction and underlying theories. The second section provides several examples of the main characteristics of this innovative instructional method and application. The third section discusses qualifications of teachers designated to deliver sheltered instruction and implications for staff development and classroom organization issues. The fourth section provides recommendations for moving beyond "sheltered" and into mainstream instructional contexts for English language learners.

Definition and Conceptual Framework

Sheltered instruction is an approach that utilizes a variety of methods designed to assist language minority (LM) students* in understanding and learning academic content (e.g., science, social studies, math, health). The primary emphasis is on teaching content, utilizing a variety of instructional techniques. Sheltered English is simply defined as:

An English language development (ELD) approach commonly referred to as sheltered English and/or sheltered content. The objective is to provide second language learners with academic content instruction through the use of specific ELD strategies that are integrated with content instruction. Instructional strategies used to accomplish this include cooperative grouping configurations, use of visuals, realia, manipulatives, and artifacts, increased wait time after a teacher has posed a question, provision for teaching prerequisite skills through a combination of specially designed instructional materials and native language support.

While sheltered instruction is not recommended as an alternative to strong primary language (L1) instruction, it is a viable means of offering instruction to LM students when the teacher speaks only English and the students have basic conversational fluency in English. Sheltered instruction usually occurs in one of the following types of settings:

- mainstream classrooms with small numbers of LM students
- multiple language classrooms (oftentimes up to six languages may be present, including English Only and Fluent English Proficient students)

---

*The term *language minority (students)* is used throughout this article to refer to students in U.S. schools who are not native speakers of English. This group includes those who are designated as limited English proficient and those who have developed some proficiency in English but are less than fully fluent. I am grateful to Tamara Lucas for the clarification and use of this term.

- designated sheltered classes, where all students are LM
- as a "transitional" class for LM students prior to entering a mainstream context where sheltered instruction is not offered.

Care must be taken in determining the optimum conditions for offering sheltered instruction. As stated earlier, it is recommended for use with students who have a working knowledge of English— i.e., the ability to verbally communicate and converse in social situations with at least an intermediate level of proficiency (Krashen, 1981). Students must be able to communicate in English as the academic content to be presented (in this case health) requires this level of fluency. Krashen (1981) and Cummins (1981) provide a set of complementary theories that contribute to a "conceptual framework" for sheltered instruction.

Approaches to Formal Language and Literacy Instruction

Traditional views of language instruction and learning focus on teaching *oral language and reading,* with an emphasis on discrete and isolated skills and rules of grammar, mainly through a phonics-based approach and basal reading instruction. This type of instruction is characterized by the use of workbooks, pencil/paper activities, and instruction that is teacher centered with little opportunity for active student engagement.

Current views toward language and literacy instruction include an emphasis on *spoken language use* and *reading and writing across the content core curricula.* This view moves beyond an emphasis on reading and isolated skills instruction to a holistic view of language and literacy that includes reading and process writing and is a response to isolated, segmented skills instruction. Current language and literacy instruction stresses function and meaning and is a pedagogy that focuses on *how* children learn and students' construction of meaning. Whole language instruction is student centered and builds on students' knowledge and understanding.

First Language Acquisition

Cummins (1981) articulates the role of first language (L1) acquisition (i.e., the nature of L1 and literacy) and the role it plays in second language acquisition. Simply put, he shows how children *acquire* rather than *learn* their first language in a natural context (i.e., engaging, communicating, talking in everyday/daily situations). He reminds us that infants acquire language in an environmental context (i.e., from family members) first through *listening* and becoming acquainted with the sounds of the language and the meanings of specific words and utterances over time.

As the child enters formal schooling, he or she has built a functional vocabulary that allows him or her to converse in a variety of contexts such as home, preschool or playgroup. The child is able to use language to ask questions, make explicit requests, gather information, etc. Upon entry into school, children begin the formal study of language and literacy.

Second Language Acquisition

Cummins (1981) stresses that students who are literate (able to speak, read and write in their first language) will be able to transfer reading and writing skills to the new language. Cummins' theories of first language acquisition are somewhat similar to Krashen's theories of second language acquisition. Krashen (1981) postulates that children acquiring a second language move through a series of stages beginning with a period of time where the student is virtually silent, looking for clues as a way of building meaning, and eventually advances to increased fluency in English language use (e.g., use of one and two word utterances, short phrases, simple sentences, etc.). At this point, naturally, mistakes may be made (as in first language acquisition) and eventually students will self-correct. Thus, the second language learner moves through a series of stages beginning with a silent period (preproduction), advancing to speech emergence, early and intermediate fluency, and, finally, full production. Ideally, sheltered instruction is introduced at the *intermediate fluency stage* as a method of instruction that supports the second language learner to full production.

First and second language acquisition theory complements the conceptual framework of whole language instruction by:

- building on what students know
- emphasizing language and literacy learning in a natural context
- sharing an approach to pedagogy that builds from the whole to the part
- de-emphasizing overt error correction and discrete skills instruction
- building meaning and students' construction of knowledge rather than emphasizing rote memorization of facts, rules of grammar and comprehension building as "direct recall"
- building the second language in a meaningful context with a focus on content and meaning
- basing teaching on how children learn and on what they need and want to learn (meaning)
- *not* administering a new set of lessons or activities to do, but approaching learning and instruction by *thinking* about how children learn.

Main Characteristics of Sheltered Instruction

Sheltered instruction is used primarily by mainstream content area teachers. It focuses on teaching academic content to LM students. This instructional approach calls for the integration of English language development strategies into the teaching of content. The following general techniques are incorporated:

- cooperative grouping
- use of visuals

- use of advance organizers
- brainstorming
- flexible groups (e.g., homogeneous/heterogeneous grouping)
- provision for teaching prerequisite skills (e.g., vocabulary, pre-teaching of vocabulary and content to be covered in a given lesson)
- use of manipulatives and artifacts to increase comprehensible input
- use of specially designed instructional materials

Several environmental features guide effective sheltered instruction (Castaneda, 1991). First, students must feel that they are allowed to think about and "theorize" about their second language (e.g., its use, application in reading and writing) in an environment where it is "OK to make a mistake." Other environmental features include the presence and acceptance of active student/student and teacher/student interaction and participation in classroom learning and related activities. This is most often achieved through the use of cooperative group tasks and student-centered rather than teacher-centered instruction. Sheltered instruction is in direct opposition to linear "top down" transmission models of education. In a sheltered environment the teacher acts as a "facilitator" of learning through the promotion of various grouping configurations, organization of learning activities and high degrees of student engagement in meaningful activities.

In a study of effective Special Alternative Instructional Programs (SAIPs), Tikunoff et al. (1991) identified three significant features at the instructional level with regard to sheltered instruction:

1. Exemplary SAIP teachers integrated principles of effective instruction with English language development. They used a mix of effective instructional practices at "various frequencies

and differently across elementary, middle/junior high and high school levels."

2. Exemplary SAIP teachers organized activities that promoted the LM students' active use of language.

3. Teachers used LM students' native languages for English language and concept development. For example, in a typical exemplary SAIP classroom, students were actively involved in their learning. In some instances students were allowed and encouraged to help and assist one another in either the first or second language. Students were grouped in a variety of ways, depending on the objectives of the lesson.

Examples of Sheltered Instruction

The following examples illustrate the use of holistic teaching strategies and active student participation in a sheltered context. This first example also illustrates the use of the students' L1 in a sheltered context. The setting is a fourth-grade classroom where the LM students had at least intermediate fluency in English.

> On this particular morning the teacher began the social studies lesson with the whole group, posing questions as she pointed to a large wall map of the United States. "Who lived here before any of the explorers?" she asked. Several students called out, "The Indians." Next, the teacher continued to build the lesson by showing the children the location of Spain. Using the map she explained the route the Spaniards used in coming to the New World.
>
> The teacher provided clear explanations, interspersed with questions. The students readily called out answers. For example, she asked, "How do you think the Indians felt when they saw the Spanish

explorers on their horses?" Different students responded, "scared," and "excited." The teacher continued to pose different questions such as, "How were the Spanish treated by the Indians?" The students called out, "like gods," and "like kings."

Next, the teacher sent a group of five students to sit with the instructional aide where they received the next portion of the lesson with clarifications and explanations provided in Armenian. The instructional aide translated and explained while the teacher continued to use shelter instruction for the remainder of the class. During this portion of the lesson the teacher had the children sit with partners to complete a number of tasks (e.g., locate Mexico and Spain in the textbook; "See if you can find Hernan Cortes' route from Spain to Mexico.") The teacher also assigned cooperative pairs to read the handout "Cortes: The conquest of Mexico."

The partners proceeded to read in a variety of ways (which were clearly decided on by the pairs). For example: One student reading while the other listened by turns; both students reading at the same time; and several pairs reading independently, without taking turns. After the students finished this activity the teacher asked, "What did the Spaniards look like?" The students responded with, "white," "red beard," and "on top of horses." The teacher proceeded to write these student responses on a large sheet of chart paper taped across the board.

This lesson segment illustrates the use of several instructional strategies that are integral pieces of a good sheltered lesson. These strategies include active participation of students; using a variety of grouping configurations, from whole group to partner pairs and back to whole group; reading and recording activities; and use of students' L1 in order to build concepts. Let us elaborate on the use of the students' primary language as an instructional technique in sheltered instruction.

While it is highly recommended that teachers not mix languages in teaching English as a second language (ESL), researchers (Tikunoff et al., 1991; Lucas and Katz, 1991) have shown that in effective sheltered classrooms, use of the students' primary language is common and serves an important role—that is, it provides increased opportunities for LM students to "access" the subject matter content being presented. It is further used to clarify concepts and build meaning. In this case, the focus is on using the students' primary language to build content, rather than on teaching language, as in ESL instruction.

The next example is taken from a high school social studies class. The class is a mainstream high school class, with a small number of LM students. The teacher has received comprehensive staff development in sheltered instruction. She provides sheltered instruction within a mainstream instructional context, using a combination of effective instructional strategies, both general and specific for LM students, along with her knowledge of first and second language acquisition.

> This discussion revolved around the Japanese-American relocation camps. The teacher began the lesson by writing the word "prejudice" on the board. She drew a large circle around the word and then asked the students to think about the word *prejudice*. "What comes to mind when you think about the word *prejudice*?" The students called out different

words (discrimination, KKK, White/Black, unjustified, racial, hate, Rodney King, religious, beatings, White supremacy, fear, inferiority, cruelty, Jim Crow, ignorance, hatred of someone) and the teacher wrote them on the board for this brainstorming activity. As the teacher wrote the various "associations" she asked the students to provide examples. Next, she instructed the students, "What I want you to do now, with a partner, is to categorize these." As the students worked in pairs the teacher began to move around to each, asking questions and clarifying. As one student discussed the terms from the brainstorming activity the partner recorded the ideas.

After the partnering activity, the teacher called the class back to the whole group and asked, "In 1942, which of these things would have applied to the Japanese?" Students returned to their pairs to discuss this. Several minutes later the teacher stated, "OK, what I'd like you to do now is come up with causes." Students continued to discuss in pairs. The next discussion centered around the categorizing activity—"What are some of the things you had trouble with?" One of the pairs (one English-speaking and one LM student) provided this response. The LM student stated that "prejudice" is both a cause and an effect, as in the case of Rodney King (Fieldnotes, Spring 1992).

Next, the teacher continued the discussion of the Japanese internment by asking the students to provide examples of the cause and effect surrounding this historical issue. The students offered input including "discrimination, violence, lack of knowledge, anger, insecurity, easy to spot as a group." Then the teacher asked, "Was there justification for relocating the Japanese?" The discussion continued as the teacher used transparencies to support the discussion.

The first transparency consisted of a view of Japan from a 1920s school text. This transparency portrayed Japan with descriptors like "modern army and navy" and "world power." After a discussion of this transparency and the view of Japan based on the 1920 U.S. text, the teacher showed a transparency of the same text, 1941 edition. This transparency portrayed Japan with descriptors like "enemy." For the next portion of the lesson the teacher had the students work in teams to draw a "symbol" of Japan for the 1990s. The students drew pictures such as "...a car running over the United States." The teacher reminded the students, "In drawing this you are showing prejudice." The students agreed.

This lesson segment is a good example of sheltered instruction in a secondary setting. The teacher used a variety of effective instructional techniques, including the use of the brainstorming activity, teacher posing questions, and the overall "back and forth" movement of the lesson from teacher directed/whole group to student/student interaction and task completion (partner pairs). LM students were partnered with English-only students. The use of visuals (transparencies) further supported the lesson. Overall, a key feature of this segment shows equal participation of the teacher and students, in that unlike "traditional" classrooms the teacher did not merely lecture to the students and do most of the talking.

Application of Sheltered Instruction

In the preceding section two examples of sheltered "segments" were presented. Next, I offer a "plan" for sheltering instruction for health education. First, I provide an overview of sheltered lesson planning in general, and then make it specific to health education.

Sheltered instruction should be viewed as a nontraditional pedagogical approach. It uses a variety of effective holistic teaching strategies coupled with knowledge of first and second language acquisition as well as activities that promote high levels of student engagement. An underlying belief that guides sheltered instruction is that all children can learn. Thus, sheltered instruction is not based on a "new" and separate set of curricula. In fact, as shown in the SAIP study, sheltered instruction is designed around grade level content area materials in a given subject. Curricula are presented in a way that makes academic knowledge, information and concepts more comprehensible. Generally teachers work in teams within their subject area or across areas. Together, they review the curricula for a given subject area and work to identify the steps identified in Figure 1.

Vocabulary is introduced within the context of the lesson. Effective vocabulary strategies include categorizing and classifying words, presenting vocabulary in context, providing simple definitions, and offering pictures and actions to reinforce meaning. A typical sheltered lesson may be planned according to the format shown in Figure 2.

Figure 1
Steps in Planning for Sheltered Instruction

- identification of key concepts
- defining measurable objectives
- designing supplementary materials and activities
- selection of methods to be used in teaching the lesson (e.g., oral discussion of lesson, brainstorming, mapping and clustering of concepts, using learning logs and journals)
- identification of key vocabulary to be covered
- identification of areas for pre-teaching
- steps to be taken in "teaching" the content and interspersed activities designed to promote high levels of student engagement
- selection of visuals and manipulatives to support concept development and build comprehensible input

---

Figure 2
Sheltered Lesson Planning Form

1. Lesson Title
2. Main Concepts (2 maximum)
3. Student Outcomes (acceptable mastery levels)
4. Contextual Clues (materials to build comprehensible input, e.g., realia, visuals, graphics, manipulatives)
5. Pre-Teaching Activities (to create background knowledge)
6. Sequence of Activities (include opportunities for student interaction)
   Lesson presentation—Sequence and list activities; indicate who is "talking," indicate type of activity (e.g., jigsaw activity, brainstorming activity, oral discussion); indicate if whole, small group or partner work along with each activity. Provide ongoing activities for large and small group work, with both teacher-directed and student-directed activities. Discussion and comprehension checks should be interspersed.
7. Comprehension Checks (can also be included in the context of the lesson and are highly recommended)

Figure 3 provides a concrete example of sheltered health planning and follows the format described.

Figure 3
Sample Sheltered Lesson on Nutrition

Lesson Title: Eating Nutritiously

Main Concepts: 1. The six food groups from the food pyramid
    2. Eating "good" foods

Student Outcomes: 1. Students will be able to identify the six food groups from the food pyramid.
    2. Students will be able to plan a well-balanced meal.

Contextual Clues: Magazines (with lots of pictures of food), transparencies depicting foods, paper plates, real food items (optional), large sheets of chart paper for graphing food groups.

Pre-Teaching: Ask each student to think about one thing that shows she or he is healthy. Have students share this information with a partner. As a whole group, list the student responses on a large sheet of chart paper labeled "Things That Make Me Healthy."

Sequence of Activities

Activity	Method	Who's Talking	Group
• healthy food	brainstorm	teacher/students	whole
• food pyramid	lecture/demo	teacher	whole
• food groups from the food pyramid	jigsaw	students	cooperative
• plan a meal	discuss/plan	students	partner pairs

Figure 3 (continued)

Comprehension Checks

Activity

Healthy Food	How would you categorize each of these foods? Why?
Food Pyramid	How much should we eat of each food group on a daily basis? (grains, fruits, vegetables, milk, meat, others [fats and oils])
Food Groups from the Food Pyramid	Name/draw a picture of the six food groups.
Plan a Meal	How much should we eat of each food group in a well-balanced meal? Tell about the foods you selected.
Closure	Working in small groups, create a graph of the most favorite and least favorite foods. Pull from the food groups selected in the Plan a Meal activity.

It should be noted that this type of planning must be ongoing within a given department or grade level. This format is recommended for use as a *planning guide only* and should be "talked out" by the cooperating teachers as they begin to implement this type of instruction.

Qualifications of Teachers: Implications for Staff Development

The terms *staff development, professional development, inservice* and *assistance* may be used interchangeably (Tikunoff et al., 1991). Staff development usually occurs at the "inservice" level—that is, activities and processes are designed to improve the teaching and instructional skills (and presumably performance) of teachers, administrators and classified staff. The design and successful implementation of effective staff development for educators who are already placed in schools is a difficult task to accomplish. Research has shown time and again that the one-shot, afterschool model of "inservice" education simply doesn't work. In the case of preparing teachers to work with LM students this is especially true. In this section, I will review the necessary qualifications for teachers providing sheltered instruction and the implications for staff development.

What are the necessary qualifications and competencies for teachers who plan and deliver content area/sheltered instruction for LM students? Several general principles must be investigated. The first principle states that teachers have the necessary opportunities to "reflect critically" on their own notions and beliefs regarding the education of LM students. Staff development opportunities must move beyond transmitting information in a "top-down" approach. A major shortcoming of staff development for inservice and veteran teachers is the lack of opportunities for discussion and reflection on what works, what doesn't work, and what "I" would like to try out. Opportunities for process work (e.g., thinking about how we think about teaching, learning, our students, necessary competencies for students and how to "teach" them) are necessary activities that must be directly connected to any staff development effort.

The second principle for effective staff development in LM issues relates to teachers' beliefs and attitudes about students in general and LM students specifically. As teachers and administrators begin to reflect critically and analyze their notions toward learning and instruction, they will begin to bridge notions about the students with whom they are working, planning programs for, etc. What belief systems (about students) guide curriculum and instruction? Do our belief systems and notions differ for various students? Why? The overall objective of this principle states that educators must reflect on their own beliefs, biases, preconceived notions, prejudices—hopefully, moving through a set of "paradigm shifts" which can never be forced, but, (potentially) may occur over time (Castaneda, 1992).

The third principle which should guide any serious staff development effort addresses the issue of *time and institutional commitment*. Effective staff development efforts should be planned and implemented with teacher, administrator, support staff and community input. Research shows that effective training of teachers should be ongoing (in terms of training, reflection, in-class practice of strategies covered, more reflection, revisiting of strategies tried, revamping strategies) throughout the academic year. Showers (1980, 1983) refers to this type of interaction as building "communities of teachers who continuously engage in the study of their craft." In a recent study of staff development efforts for mainstream English-only speaking teachers, these salient features emerged (Castaneda, 1992):

- Training processes called for active involvement of participants.
- While the theory and instructional strategies were presented, they were modeled in the actual delivery by the trainers.
- Trainers taught and modeled group processing skills designed to promote active student engagement and face-to-face interaction.
- After a theory or method was "taught" it was modeled and analyzed by the trainees.
- Trainees had opportunities to explore alternative approaches to classroom organization (e.g., self-contained, teaming, cross-age grouping, schoolwide scheduling).
- Training was tied into actual classroom practice through peer-coaching activities. Trainers served as peer coaches and (upon

invitation from the teacher) observed the trainee as she or he implemented the training into teaching.
- Peer coaches (upon invitation from the classroom teacher) modeled lessons for the trainees in order to connect theories and methods (covered in training) to practice.

In terms of general competencies which should guide staff development efforts for teachers preparing to shelter content subject matter the following are recommended.

First and second language acquisition theory:
- knowledge of first and second language acquisition theory and tie-in to practice; (Basic Interpersonal Communication Skills [BICS] and Cognitive Academic Language Proficiency [CALPs])
- understanding of similarities and differences in teaching ESL, ELD, Sheltered Content Instruction
- application of first and second language acquisition principles to content area/academic instruction
- ability to prepare and deliver specially designed academic lessons
- historical and current theories

Effective instructional/organizational practices:
- organization of instruction based on a variety of instructional configurations (e.g., whole group, small group, partner pairs)
- cooperative grouping practices
- use/integration of various learning modalities in curriculum and instruction
- literacy (reading and writing) across the content core curricula
- holistic instructional strategies
- team teaching, cross-grade grouping, schoolwide scheduling
- peer coaching

Culture:
- diversity issues
- generic understanding of culture (sociocultural/sociolinguistic perspectives)
- the nature of culture within a theoretical and applied context
- culture as communication
- communication/interaction in school and community contexts

Staff development efforts in the SAIP study (Tikunoff, et al., 1991) covered the types of competencies outlined here. However, special attention must always be paid to the needs of the local school site in terms of determining needs and planning appropriate staff development activities. In the SAIP study, overall, teachers played an important role in the areas of leadership, decision making and input into the areas of professional development. Teacher involvement must continue to grow—as a way of addressing the local needs. Finally, effective staff development efforts at the SAIP sites offered ongoing support and incentives for the teacher participants. First, teachers were "invited" (rather than required) to participate in the professional development efforts. Second, teachers were not asked to teach all day and then attend an after school inservice meeting. Instead, teachers were supported with released time (usually by obtaining substitute teachers) to attend the training sessions during the work day. Third, when after-school or Saturday training sessions were offered, teachers were paid an honorarium for their attendance.

Moving Beyond Sheltered Instruction

What will it take to address the needs of ethnolinguistically diverse students once they enter mainstream English-only contexts? What happens to students once they leave specialized environments designed to address their specific academic and linguistic needs (as in bilingual and sheltered classes)? In this section I discuss issues surrounding the effective education of LM students once they have left specialized environments. This discussion moves beyond appropriate methodology and theory (although these still play a significant role), and, instead, looks at ways of thinking about and "doing" teaching and learning.

One of the major concerns for all educators has to do with *thinking*. How do we think about teaching? How do we think about our students? How do we think about learning? What are our expectations of our students? The following research offers a possible avenue for planning, implementing and revisiting appropriate, successful educational experiences for all students. With ongoing reflection and analysis we can address the particular concerns of those LM students who are expected to function in "regular" English mainstream contexts.

In a recent study of an effective staff development effort aimed at addressing the needs of high school LM students and their English-only teachers, it was documented that teachers began to change their views, expectations, and perhaps "paradigms." Yet, an explicit attempt to change the teachers' thinking about their methodologies, guiding beliefs and theory about their work with LM students was never intended (Castaneda, 1992). However, for this particular staff development effort, several significant features emerged that may have contributed to the shift. First, teachers were provided with ongoing, consistent opportunities to "try out" new strategies in class, often with the opportunity to "reflect, react, and (in some instances) rethink" their delivery of a certain lesson, or the general outcome. This reflection time often occurred individually or in consultation with a team partner or peer coach. Reflection was ongoing and teachers had a variety of built-in opportunities, both in the staff development and teaching contexts.

For example, teacher teams had one period a day of daily planning time to discuss methods tried, reactions to lessons and student reaction (e.g., involvement, engagement). Another feature that supported the teachers' "thinking" had to do with the activities during staff development that promoted teachers' reading, discussion, critical analyses of recent theory, and pedagogy surrounding effective curricula and instruction both in general and specifically for LM students. I believe that, given the opportunity to critically think, reflect, analyze and apply to real classroom situations, teachers will be able to utilize this information. With regard to learning, instruction, literacy and critical thinking, they will make appropriate, informed, decisions about curricula and instruction for their students. For the teachers who have not had prior training in the areas of language acquisition, culture and methodology, this will be critical for their development as competent practitioners. However, development and reflection should not end here for any educator.

In sum, the needs of LM students are clear. And the types of pedagogical approaches and theoretical underpinnings associated with their education may also contribute to the educational experience of other students. Moving beyond sheltered English will involve a variety of shifts, and must be supported with ongoing staff development and an emphasis on teachers' thinking about their own pedagogy. This thinking will involve planning, implementation and analysis, as educators take into account their students' diverse ways of learning, acquiring and using knowledge. Addressing the needs of LM students should focus on issues that reach beyond a new set of curricula or program—it must involve a constant look at pedagogy, theory, reflection and overall implications for practice.

References

Castaneda, L. V. 1991. The social organization of communication and interaction in SAIP classrooms and the nature of competent classroom membership. Paper presented at the annual meeting of the American Educational Research Association, Chicago.

Castaneda, L. V. 1992. Alternative visions of practice: An exploratory study of peer coaching, sheltered content, cooperative instruction, and mainstream subject matter teachers. Proceedings of paper presented at the National Research Symposium on Limited English Proficient Students Issues, August 12-14, 1992. Washington, DC.

Cummins, J. 1981. The role of primary language development in promoting educational success for language minority students. In *Schooling and language minority students: A theoretical framework*. Los Angeles, CA: Evaluation, Dissemination and Assessment Center, California State University Los Angeles.

Krashen, S. D. 1981. Bilingual education and second language acquisition theory. In *Schooling and language minority students: A theoretical framework*. Los Angeles, CA: Evaluation, Dissemination and Assessment Center, California State University Los Angeles.

Lucas, T., and A. Katz. 1991. The role of students' native languages in Exemplary SAIPs. Paper presented at the annual meeting of the American Educational Research Association, Chicago, April.

Showers, J. B. 1983. *Power in staff development through research on training*. Alexandria, VA: Association for Supervision and Curriculum Development.

Showers, J. B. 1980. Improving inservice training: The messages of research. *Educational Leadership* 37:379-385.

Tikunoff, W. J., B. A. Ward, D. van Broekhuizen, M. Romero, L. V. Castaneda, T. Lucas and A. Katz. 1991. *A descriptive study of significant features of exemplary special alternative instructional programs*. Los Alamitos, CA: The Southwest Regional Laboratory.

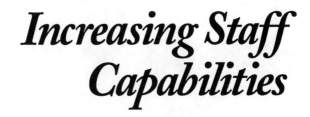

Increasing Staff Capabilities

Chapter 12

Shifting the Dominant Paradigm: A Challenge for Administrators

Maria Natera, EdD

> The only choice for an institution is between man-
> agement and mismanagement.... Whether it is being
> done right or not will determine largely whether the
> enterprise will survive and prosper or decline and
> ultimately fail.
>
> —Peter Drucker

Ten years ago, the National Commission on Excellence in Education concluded that due to the low performance of our schools, we were "a nation at risk." Although the effort to reform the schools predated the commission's report, the document served to provide some additional intensity. In the last thirty years, we have seen three waves of educational reform in this country. Our schools are in the midst of what appears to be the third major wave of reform in the attempt to provide quality education for all children.

The first wave came in the late sixties with the Elementary and Secondary Educational Act (ESEA), educational amendments under the leadership of President Johnson. In this first wave there were over sixty federal and state laws directing us to educate all children including the poor, the physically challenged, children of color, migrant students and the non-English speaking. The second wave of reform came in the late 1970s and focused on strengthening the curriculum and setting higher standards for students and teachers.

We are now in the third wave, which is challenging the structure of the public schools. Restructuring philosophy encourages site-based management and changing the school in any way possible that will benefit the students and improve their academic performance. It encourages schools to collaborate with community agencies. The belief is that through this collaboration and other restructuring strategies, students will begin to realize they are valuable resources for their community, and this will empower them as active and engaged learners and citizens.

Most schools that have been involved in the restructuring movement have developed sound curricular goals and objectives, and they constantly strive for effectiveness and efficiency. However, they perform less well in communities characterized by ethnic and linguistic diversity, particularly in the building of trusting relationships among key faculty, staff, students, parents and the rest of the community. Could this be because multiethnic communities have become more and more isolated from their local schools and other public agencies that are supposed to serve them? Or could it be that issues of equity and diversity are typically not part of the restructuring dialogue?

The last ten years of intense reform and restructuring among our schools produced self-examination and efforts at renewal. These efforts have failed to reach the multiethnic student populations with any significance. Presently "at-risk" students are still comprised of a disproportionate number of students of color, students with limited English proficiency, migrant students, the poor and the physically challenged.

I and my associates have worked extensively as educational and organizational development consultants with dozens of public schools in California. In almost every school we met people concerned about inequities and the failure of certain aspects of the restructuring efforts to address the needs of particular students. In general, however, we discovered that issues of equity and diversity were typically not part of the restructuring dialogue.

Addressing Issues of Equity and Diversity

California Tomorrow, a nonprofit organization dedicated to promoting equity and diversity in California, conducted a study of the schools that had received restructuring grants from the California Department of Education. One of their initial findings was that school administrators and staff were not engaging in open dialogue on the issues of "equity and diversity."

In our meetings with administrators, teachers and other school staff, as well as with parents and other community members in various school districts, our observations paralleled the findings of California Tomorrow. While the lack of communication wasn't as evident when we met with school personnel, we found parents and community members frustrated by the lack of attention given to their pressing needs. This failure of the restructuring movement to address issues of equity and diversity, the isolation of communities of color and the ever shrinking educational funding and resources has caused bitter alienation in some schools.

In their report, California Tomorrow attributed the lack of discussion of equity and diversity issues to some of the following factors. Others are the author's additions.

Dominant paradigm. Raising issues of equity or diversity goes against the existing dominant paradigm which advocates for a colorblind approach. The colorblind approach de-emphasizes differences and advocates for a universal, generic system of education as a strategy for ensuring all children equal access to a strong curriculum. People who have specific expertise and experience in the issues facing the various cultural and ethnic groups have felt that their contribution was undervalued. The unspoken message is "we do not value your input." They tend to be excluded from the dialogue because they are not invited to the discussion, or their voices are discounted because they have a lower status within the school community.

Discussing difficult issues. Issues of equity and diversity are difficult to discuss. They can be threatening and even explosive. School staff often lack the skills, the appropriate forum or trained facilitators to conduct nonthreatening discussions and to address these issues. An example of a difficult issue that is beginning to receive attention is student sexual harassment. Some superintendents and principals who have been approached by consultants from the Gender Equity Unit of the California Department of Education offering free preventative education have responded by saying that training would only make the problem worse. Yet, Senator Hart's Bill (SB 1930) on student-to-student sexual harassment makes it possible for a fourth grader to be expelled from school if he or she engages in "sexual harassment" of another student. If the schools do not set clear guidelines, a student might say or do something unacceptable without realizing that his or her behavior is considered sexual harassment. The "let's not talk about it" policy keeps the problem in denial and our students suffer the consequences.

Lack of leadership expertise. The people in leadership roles in schools attempting to restructure often lack the expertise, experience or data which would allow them to raise the issues of equity and diversity. Additionally, they may need training in management techniques that could enable them to be more inclusive of key staff and the community. For example, when Total Quality Management is not practiced, leaders at a school may not include key staff, parents and community members in the dialogue. Yet when the student outcomes are analyzed, few mention the exclusion of these crucial participants.

Lack of research benefit. The restructuring dialogue does not include and consequently does not benefit from the extensive research on multicultural education, bilingual education, language development theory and other key issues related to the education of students from diverse ethnic backgrounds.

Increased alienation of communities of color. Increasingly, our world is characterized by rapid change. Managers face the difficult task of having to prepare for change rather than being passively swept along by it. The rapid growth of linguistically and ethnically diverse populations in California and other states has placed some schools in a Catch-22 cycle. School administrators and teachers watch their communities rapidly changing. This rapid change often takes place without the school and the community engaging in any kind of meaningful dialogue. New community members and the future employers of their students do not feel part of the school community and therefore have no loyalty to it. By the time school officials try to communicate with students, parents, new community members and businesses, the community has become alienated from the schools. This kind of Catch-22/nondialogue cycle tends to increase the numbers of at-risk students academically and socially. It perpetuates the dominant paradigm.

Additionally, in communities characterized by rapid change and poverty, alienation is compounded by other related problems such as violence, drugs and family distress. The schools naturally feel helpless. Although schools can't solve all of these social problems, neither can they turn their backs on them. The challenge faced by school administrators is to shift the paradigm and the nondialogue cycle and engage in open communication, build trust and provide leadership in the community.

Paradigm Shifting Through the Institutionalization of Equity and Diversity

Administrators need to institutionalize equity and diversity; it should be an integral part of the restructuring dialogue. Strategies need to be designed to eliminate unequal expectations and treatment of the poor, the physically challenged, children of color and limited English speaking students. These strategies need to become accepted features in the operation of schools in order for them to become institutionalized. When physically challenged children, the poor, the non-English speaking children and children of color are in schools where they feel physically *and* emotionally safe, are intellectually challenged and are experiencing successful outcomes, it will be clear that these schools have institutionalized equity and diversity.

In order to get closer to shifting the dominant paradigm and institutionalizing equity and diversity in our schools, we recommend that:

- Issues of equity and diversity become an integral part of the restructuring goal. We assert that ultimately we are all seeking unity and inclusion.
- All schools be staffed by a richly diverse multiracial and multilingual faculty.
- Schools engage in deliberate efforts to facilitate and create dialogue about the specific needs and issues facing the particular ethnic and linguistic groups who comprise their student populations.

- Due to difficult issues and the fear of excess conflict, a skilled facilitator be hired or otherwise secured for facilitating meetings where issues of equity and diversity will be discussed.
- A major emphasis be placed on professional development in the areas of diversity and cross-cultural communication, and that there be follow-up to professional development, with opportunities for administrators, teachers, students and parents to share their collective knowledge and experience with each other.
- School personnel have access to and be encouraged to use the extensive research and literature available on educating children from multiethnic backgrounds, including the social issues that affect their specific communities.
- The central concern of the school be to develop whole human beings and go beyond academic outcomes. This extends the curriculum to include self-esteem, self-knowledge and respect for diversity.

Paradigm Shifting through Total Quality Management

According to W. Edward Deming, who has developed the Total Quality Management (TQM) philosophy, quality is defined by the client or customer. In TQM, the whole system is devoted to continuous improvement at every step of the process. Managers empower and reward workers who report failures in quality or suggest improvements. In the case of schools, managers also encourage students and their families to give this kind of input. Managers recognize that workers are in a position to know the most about their work, and manage not through fear, but by helping to design and improve a system in which all workers can succeed. Many educators are now striving to apply this philosophy to their schools.

We believe that the TQM emphasis on bringing everyone up to mastery levels may be helpful because it requires the institutional support and culture to sustain it. In other words, which practices and institutional supports will best help all children learn? Mastery of learning and a focus on quality are two pieces that fit together to make a successful and healthy learning environment.

- The TQM school has people of color and community members as key planners and in key leadership roles.
- In TQM, people who have specific expertise and experience in the issues facing the various ethnic, cultural and linguistic groups contribute to the dialogue as equal and valued participants.
- A TQM school looks at how well the various subgroups of children are doing. Quality is defined by the customer, i.e., the students and their families.
- A TQM school is staffed by a richly diverse multiracial and multilingual faculty. This way all workers can be productive and feel pride in their work. Children in mainstream schools are also entitled to a rich and diverse faculty in order to be prepared to live in a diverse and global world.

Paradigm Shifting Through a Comprehensive School Health Program

The central issue of this book is how to make comprehensive health education more relevant to our multiethnic student population. We see an opportunity for health educators to help shift the dominant paradigm in the schools. After all, one cannot implement a comprehensive school health program without understanding the needs, aspirations, priorities and values of the students, families and communities that will benefit from health education services. The need for an integrated school and community approach is being rediscovered as an effective strategy to promote the well-being of children. Articulation of a shared vision for the health of children is an opportunity for schools to communicate with their clients.

The fact that more school and community health educators are working together to protect and improve the health of students is a double benefit. Both of these institutions are crucial systems in the lives of students. The concept of the comprehensive school health program includes not only comprehensive health education but also school health services, the school health environment, integrated efforts of school and community agencies, the physical education program, food services, counseling and psychology programs, and programs to protect and improve the health of faculty and staff. This affords us a great opportunity to be part of a true partnership that will benefit all students.

It is encouraging to see the many coalitions that are being formed to support and improve school health programs. Even more encouraging is that this strategy seems to promote inclusion of all clients in the decision-making process. This asserts that it is not schools alone that will finally make a difference, but schools, students, their families and the whole community, working together.

Chapter 13

Staff Development for Multicultural Competency

Loren B. Bensley, Jr., EdD, CHES

B eginning teachers are often of the opinion that all students should be treated the same, regardless of color, religion or ethnic background. In other words, the fair thing to do is show neither favoritism nor bias in their relationships with students. However, it is not long before they realize this is impossible. They may find that a Mexican American who speaks broken English needs more attention than others in the class. Likewise, an African American, who is rebellious and defiant as a result of struggling with his or her identity in a predominantly White school, deserves extra attention and time. As a result, a difference in treatment emerges. Realization that all students cannot be treated the same becomes even clearer when discussing various individual health practices dictated by religious and cultural beliefs. For instance, the health practices of the Islamic culture as told by an immigrant from Saudi Arabia, although different, can be fascinating, and the interest generated by other students often results in that person being the center of attention. It is through events like these, that teachers begin to realize that if they teach in a way they consider fair (all students are the same), they are actually, in the words of James Banks, "denying them an equal chance to succeed" (Banks, cited in Corner, 1984).

American education has a long history of serving diverse groups made up of generations of immigrants, Native Americans and migrants. Unfortunately, these culturally diverse groups have not always been given the attention needed. As a result of discrimination and lack of sensitivity and understanding, educational inequality has resulted. This does not mean everyone must be treated the same, but they must have a chance for equal education. The purpose of this chapter is to explore why it is important that teachers be trained in delivering culturally relevant health education. This includes the role of pre- and inservice programs in preparing health education teachers.

In order to achieve this purpose, the following issues of professional preparation and inservice training will be explored:

- Exploring the importance of teacher competencies in delivering multiethnic health education.
- Understanding the ethnographic profiles of minorities: language, values and beliefs, health status and access to health care.
- Understanding the health status of four subcultures: African Americans, Asian Americans, Hispanics and Native Americans. What do health educators, administrators and policymakers need to know in order to design and implement culturally relevant programs?
- The role of universities in preparing culturally sensitive teachers of health education.
- How health education teachers can be inserviced to become culturally literate and skilled in teaching multiethnic students.

The Importance of Teacher Competencies in Delivering Multiethnic Health Education

The democratic principles and traditions of American education have not evolved without controversy. Examples of discriminatory practices are rampant in the classrooms and public schools. Immigrant children were looked upon as inferior and in some cases were denied equal educational opportunities in the schools that were supported by taxes paid by their parents. Stereotyping was typical for individuals different from Anglo Americans. Unfortunately, some teachers' attitudes and values reflected this in the classroom. There is no better example of this than the segregation of African Americans. It took the United States Supreme Court's *Brown v. Board of Education* groundbreaking decision in 1954 to desegregate schools. Today our classrooms are integrated with individuals of various ethnic backgrounds, religious beliefs and languages, representing a variety of customs and values.

Health education teachers need to acknowledge the cultural diversity that exists in their classrooms. This diversity will continue through the 1990s, and, by the year 2000, it is predicted that one-third of our students will be members of the Asian-American, African-American, Hispanic or Native-American cultures. "Recent reports have noted that in 25 out of 26 of the largest urban school systems, minority students outnumber White students, thus making White students the nation's newest minority group" (Banks, cited in Davidman, 1990).

In order for health educators to effectively teach and relate to all children, they must have three essential qualities. They must be as free and unbiased as possible and open to continuing self-examination; they must honor and value cultural alternatives such as language, beliefs, values and behaviors; and they must feel that a multicultural orientation will benefit them as individuals as well as enhance their ability to be effective teachers (Hilliard, cited in Hunter, 1974).

All teachers bring to school their personal values and attitudes, which may or may not be free of stereotypes or bias toward other individuals or groups. When this occurs, the teacher will not be able to understand or relate to his or her students in a fair and positive way. Unless all educators learn to value difference and view it as a resource for learning, neither majority nor minority groups will experience the best teaching and learning situations to prepare them to live effectively with people of many cultures (Pine and Hilliard, 1989).

Health educators must honor and value cultural differences such as language, beliefs, values and behaviors in order to gain respect from their students. They must also have these qualities to be able to design effective curricula and implement culturally relevant teaching strategies. A person's cultural differences are unique. When this is not acknowledged, students will feel prejudice and ridicule, which can easily destroy their self-esteem. Recognizing students' cultural differences and encouraging pride in themselves and their culture can be a powerful tool in teaching healthy lifestyles. Furthermore, the teacher's credibility is enhanced by his or her willingness to honor and value cultural differences.

Teachers must realize the benefits of a multiethnic orientation. Having a background in understanding various cultures will help them be more effective teachers. Those who close their eyes and ears to the need for an understanding of the backgrounds of the children they teach are setting themselves up for failure. The teacher's attitude toward teaching in a multiethnic setting is the first consideration in meeting the personal and professional challenge that can lead to satisfaction and confidence in his or her teaching abilities. Preparing oneself to teach in a multiethnic classroom demands an open mind and a positive attitude towards the beliefs and values of all groups.

The National Council for the Accreditation of Teacher Education (NCATE) recognizes that teacher education programs have a responsibility to prepare teacher candidates to understand and be able to teach multiethnic populations. The *1992 Standards, Procedures, and Policies for the Accreditation of Professional Education Units*, states that professional studies for the preparation of teachers should include cultural influences on learning. This includes the understanding and application of appropriate strategies for individual learning needs, especially for culturally diverse and exceptional populations. The specific standards for the accreditation of professional preparation programs for school health educators lists competencies that must be met so that prospective health educators will be able to select methods and media best suited to implement program plans for specific learners; determine the availability of information, personnel, time and equipment needed to implement programs for a given audience; and evaluate the worth and applicability of resource material. (Robinson, Ames and Olsen, 1991). This supports the need for teacher education programs that design their curricula to assist students in developing attitudes and skills relevant to multiethnic groups.

This is necessary due to the fact that school health education has become an important channel for primary prevention programs because of its mission and mandated attendance policy. This is especially true in the case of providing health education for youth from ethnically diverse backgrounds, since poverty and discrimination often leave other community socializing agencies unable to provide primary prevention. Therefore, the role of the health educator in serving the students of multiethnic origin becomes even more crucial (Centers for Disease Control and Prevention, 1992).

Understanding Ethnographic Profiles of Minorities

Effective health instruction cannot be accomplished without training in cross-cultural communication and methodology. The classroom teacher needs to be able to relate cognitive information and skill development to the complexities of multiethnic values, beliefs, traditions and practices. To do this, the teacher must be knowledgeable and sensitive to various cultural groups.

To be an effective health educator, one must understand the values, beliefs, traditions and practices of different cultures and the effect that these have on the way they experience health. "For example, in some cultural groups health and illness are believed to be determined by the balance or imbalance of spiritual or supernatural forces, rather than by biological, behavioral or environmental factors alone" (Gonzalez et al., 1991). Health educators' nonjudgmental understanding of these different beliefs and practices, as well as how they differ from their own, will greatly affect their ability to develop curricula and plan teaching strategies to help them relate to multiethnic students.

In attempting to understand cultures, it is necessary to identify the factors that constitute a culture. There are three aspects of all cultures which make them unique. Furthermore, each of these factors can play a significant role in determining the health practices of multiethnic students. These factors—language, religion, and values and beliefs—are discussed briefly for the purpose of understanding the makeup of a culture, as well as the specifics of each factor which may have an impact on health status or health practices.

Language

The language of a group provides a common bond for individuals. For example, the dialect or language used in the right situation can provide the individual immediate acceptance or credibility (Frazee and Johnson, 1993). Language is probably the single most important cultural identity that bonds groups of individuals together. Often students will enter school with English as a second language. As a result, their understanding of the spoken as well as written word is often confused. It is important that the health educator recognize the difficulties experienced by these students in understanding the content of health education.

In addition to the language, there are oral communication skills that sometimes are unique to certain cultures. For example, in addressing Asian Americans, direct eye contact may be considered extremely rude. Asian Americans may not ask questions of persons in authority because they consider this to be disrespectful (Frazee and Johnson, 1993). In communicating with African Americans, it is important not to try to adopt "Black English" because this may be viewed as insulting. When communicating with Hispanic Americans, formal titles are extremely important as an indication of respect (Frazee and Johnson, 1993).

With Native Americans, direct eye contact often is considered disrespectful. Handshakes are very much a part of Native American culture and are considered an important symbolic gesture. Another example of communication problems with Native Americans is that some English words and concepts do not exist in Indian languages or are not easily translatable (Frazee and Johnson, 1993). In addition, the health educator must realize the content of health education often is technical and utilizes a variety of scientific words and terms. Language can, therefore, be a severe handicap for the student who is not familiar with the English language.

It would be helpful if the health education teacher could speak the language of the learner. This would greatly improve not only the communication and credibility of the teacher, but the chances of employment for beginning teachers and relocation for those who are experienced. The ability to speak Spanish would greatly enhance the teaching effectiveness of those who choose to teach in the southwestern region of the country or in large cities where there are Spanish-speaking populations.

Religion

Religion is another important factor in separating cultures. Some religions dictate the behavior of groups by instilling beliefs and values that may be harmful to health. Thus, with certain cultures, health education may be contrary to the religious beliefs of learners. Not recognizing these differences would be insensitive and possibly alienate the student. (Gonzalez, cited in Frazee and Johnson, 1993) For example, Native Americans may believe in the medicine man and his practice of herbal medicine. If Native Americans are part of a health education class, the teacher should become familiar with the practice of Native American medicine, which includes the use of herbal medicine, dances, spiritual healing and other traditions used by the medicine man. Another example of the influence of religion, which may contradict healthful practices, would be the use of peyote and other drugs which are acceptable among Native Americans as part of religious ceremonies.

Islam is a rapidly growing religion practiced by many immigrants in the United States. Most of what is known about Islamic health sciences has been taken from the Koran, which is the scripture book of Islam. Ghazizadeh (1992) describes the relationship between the Islamic faith and health practices by explaining that personal appearance and physical cleanliness are just as important as spiritual purity. He further states that certain prohibitions such as eating pork, drinking alcohol, gambling, abortion, adultery, incest, etc., are for the protection of the individual's and society's health and well-being. Brushing the teeth is recommended before each of the five daily prayers practiced by Muslims. In Islamic faith, education is an important subject, and, therefore, Muslims are encouraged not to be ashamed and to seek answers to their questions concerning human sexuality. "Prophet Mohammed answered all questions concerning sex, indicating that there is no shyness in the matter of religion" (Ghazizadeh, 1992).

These are only a few examples of the interrelationship between religion and health beliefs and practices. Assuming that there is a connection between health and religion, it is important that health educators understand religious practices as they affect a person's health. This understanding can result from asking questions of students, their parents and other community resources, or from reading about the nature of health as it relates to different religions.

Values and Beliefs

The values and beliefs of a culture are often dictated by religion. There are also values and beliefs which stem from other aspects of the culture. These may involve political philosophy, economics, social customs and family traditions. The health education teacher must realize that cultural values may be very difficult to change. Furthermore, values are often family centered and could become controversial if the health educator is not sensitive to cultural beliefs. For example, in some cultures health is viewed as a family or religious responsibility, rather than just of the individual. As previously mentioned, those of the Islamic faith value health highly, and this is reflected in their daily life.

Certain cultures may value folk medicine which has been handed down from one generation to another. The health educator may find the values and beliefs in nontraditional medicine difficult to accept. This is when sensitivity becomes important to help the health educator accept values of nontraditional medicine practiced by these students. To disagree or to argue with the student regarding nontraditional beliefs could erode the teacher's credibility.

As mentioned earlier, family values can influence positive health practices. One example is the Hispanic culture which values the family unit. Responsibility of caring for one another and maintaining family loyalty is a positive factor in the mental health of Hispanics.

Attitude toward education is also a factor that can influence the success of health education. For example Asian Americans place a high value on education and are extremely goal oriented. This particular cultural value explains the high achievement of many immigrants from Cambodia, Vietnam, Japan and Korea. Likewise, some cultures value the opportunity for free education that is offered in the United States. This being the case, there is a tendency for parents to urge their children to achieve in school. This is especially true with newly arrived immigrants.

According to Frazee and Johnson (1993), the health education teacher must realize that "values that one culture views as positive may be considered undesirable or threatening in another. Values commonly found in the United States may be inappropriate to other cultures. Simply exposing students to a new idea or practice will not automatically result in adoption if that idea or practice conflicts with their values. There is a natural tendency for people to be culture bound, to assume that their values, customs, and behaviors are admirable, sensible, and right. Cross-cultural health education presents a special challenge because it requires the teacher to work with students without making judgments as to the superiority of one set of values over another."

Leslie and Mikanowicz (1992) identify the relationship of cultural values to teaching health education. Strategies can be adapted to assist individuals in their health maintenance such as:

- The health education curricula should be consistent with the cultural values of the population, and should accentuate and enforce representative community diversity and resources.
- The curricula should contain information based on the individual cultural values of the representative groups.
- Teaching strategies should promote open communication and incorporate terminology that is reflective, warm and sensitive to the values of the target population.

Access to Health Care

Most minorities do not have access to health care. This is one of the reasons for the high rates of premature mortality and excess morbidity among minority groups. There are three barriers to health care for minorities: physical access, economic factors and acceptability of services.

Physical access refers to barriers that interfere with availability of the care. This would include unusually long distances that would have to be traveled to receive health care, the cost for public transportation or services that would be available when needed.

Economic factors are the inability to pay for services. It is a known fact that in general, within minority groups there is a higher rate of those with little or no health insurance. As a result, fewer visits are made for health services. Furthermore, some providers may be unwilling to provide services when they know it may be unlikely they will be paid.

Acceptability of health care, or care that is user friendly, is the third factor that inhibits access to health care for multiethnic populations. Refugees and immigrants may have language difficulties which may cause a delay in seeking health care. Some other factors that may cause a lack of acceptability of health care include lack of knowledge of services, feelings of prejudice or discrimination by health care providers, intimidation of patient by health care providers or the bureaucracy of health services (Michigan Department of Public Health, 1988).

Health Status of Multiethnic Groups

Of special importance to the health educator are the various health problems associated with multiethnic groups. It is important to briefly address the specific health problems of different cultures as they relate to the provision of health education. As already discussed, health problems can be related to religious practices, cultural beliefs and values, and access to health care. In addition, socioeconomic factors, housing conditions, preventive medicine and health promotion also play a factor in the health of all cultures. Taking these into consideration, a brief discussion of health behaviors and problems of four ethnic groups will be explored. Understanding health problems of various ethnic groups is a must for the health educator.

African Americans

Life expectancy for African Americans in the United States is less than that of the total population. The discrepancy is approximately five years. There are several theories regarding this discrepancy, of which socioeconomic and environmental reasons are most commonly subscribed to. In the following examples, Frazee and Johnson (1993) identify differences in the health status of African Americans compared to other populations.

Statistics show that African-American men die from strokes at a much higher rate than men in the total population. Deaths due to coronary heart disease are higher for African-American women than for White women. African-American men experience a higher rate of cancer than White men, and diabetes is 33 percent more common among African Americans than Whites. Infant mortality rate is twice as high among African-American babies during the first year of life. Two causes of mortality which occur in much greater numbers among African Americans than the rest of the population are those related to homicide and HIV/AIDS. For example, African-American men have a 1 in 21 chance of being murdered, while African-American women are more than four times as likely to be homicide victims as White women. The rate of AIDS among African Americans is more than three times that of Whites.

Other health problems are more common among African Americans than the total population. Overweight is a problem for 44 percent of African-American women age twenty and older, compared to 27 percent for all women. Adolescent pregnancy is a major problem among the African-American population. The African-American teenage girl is approximately three times more likely to give birth than a White girl. Fifty-three percent of all Black youth are born to single mothers. Furthermore, a Black infant is twice as likely as a White infant to die before age one.

Asian Americans

Asian Americans are the fastest growing minority group in the United States today. The number of Asian Americans grew 108 percent from 1980 to 1990. Asian Americans generally live in the western part of the United States, with California being a major population center (Centers for Disease Control and Prevention, 1992). Unlike African Americans, health status and health problems of Asians cannot be ascribed to any particular socioeconomic or environmental cause.

According to Frazee and Johnson (1993), two infectious diseases are more prevalent among immigrants of Asian and Pacific Islander subgroups than the total population. These are tuberculosis and hepatitis B. This could be due to the fact that tuberculosis is still the leading cause of death in some Asian countries, and, as a result, has become a serious problem in some Asian communities in the United States. Among the risk factors, the greatest concern among Asians is smoking. As pointed out by Frazee and Johnson (1993), "smoking rates among men are 92 percent for Laotians, 71 percent for Cambodians, and 65 percent for Vietnamese, compared to 30 percent for the overall American population."

Hispanics

Individuals classified as Hispanics may be identified as Mexican Americans, Chicanos, Spanish Americans, Latin Americans, Puerto Ricans, Cubans, Guatemalans and Salvadorans (Gonzalez, cited in Baruth and Manning, 1992). Of those considered Hispanics, Mexican Americans considerably outnumber all others. One out of sixteen people in the United States in 1980 was of Hispanic origin (Baruth and Manning, 1992).

The health status of Hispanics can be related to socioeconomic conditions as well as the lack of access to health care. Frazee and Johnson (1993) list several health conditions of the Hispanic culture. Leading causes of death among Hispanics are unintentional injuries, homicide, chronic liver disease, cirrhosis and HIV/AIDS. "In the case of AIDS, Hispanics rate nearly three times higher than non-Hispanic Whites, with rates among Puerto Rican born Hispanics as much as seven times higher." The incidence of AIDS among Hispanic women is about eight times higher than among non-Hispanic women and the rate for HIV infection is over six times higher for non-Hispanic children. Diabetes is also a special problem among Mexican Americans, as is overweight, which is common among Mexican-American women.

Native Americans

Native Americans are the smallest defined minority group in the United States. Although they are few in number, they consist of many nations that speak about 220 different languages (Baruth and Manning, 1992). Frazee and Johnson (1993), present an interesting observation of Native Americans by citing the following demographic and health facts. The Native-American population is youthful with the median age of those living in the reservation states being about age 23, as compared to over 32 for the United States population as a whole. Native Americans can be found in virtually all of the states, with a heavy concentration in the southwest. Only about one-third of Native Americans live on reservations, while about 50 percent live in urban centers.

Health problems of Native Americans can be directly related to socioeconomic conditions, including poverty and lack of education. Unfortunately, a large proportion of the population dies before age 45, which can be attributed to unintentional injuries, cirrhosis, homicide, suicide, pneumonia and complications of diabetes (Frazee and Johnson, 1993). Special health concerns among Native Americans are obesity and alcoholism, which are major risk factors for several chronic diseases. It is estimated that 75 percent of deaths due to unintentional injuries are alcohol-related. Alcohol is also a factor in homicides and suicides. Cirrhosis, which is alcohol-related, is one of two chronic diseases that afflict Native Americans more frequently than other groups. Native Americans also have a higher rate of diabetes than the general population. This could be attributed to obesity which is experienced by many individuals in this culture group.

Native Americans who live on reservations have access to health facilities and health care which is provided by the Indian Health Service. Unfortunately, many Native Americans live in urban areas where access to health care may be difficult.

When teaching health education to Native Americans, it is important to recognize the alcohol and other drug problems of this particular group. Whether this is caused by environment or social customs and traditions can be debated. Unfortunately, alcohol is a serious problem for this group and needs to be understood and addressed. The health education teacher who has Native-American learners should meet with someone from the Indian Health Services, a health educator at an Indian reservation, or the local health department to try to better understand the lifestyles and health conditions of this group.

What Health Educators Need to Know in Order to Design and Implement Culturally Relevant Programs

In addition to what has already been discussed, further information is necessary in order to establish policy, construct curricula and implement teaching strategies. In reviewing the literature, Heimlich and Van Tilburg (1987) have identified five issues viewed from the perspective of the individual of a multiethnic background. These are generic cross-cultural issues that need to be considered by educators whether they're policy-makers, administrators or teachers. The issues listed have been slightly modified by the author.

Appreciate that our beliefs are different from yours. You do not have to believe as we do, but you must appreciate the fact that our beliefs are different, and, even more than that, you must learn to live with those beliefs. You may not have to accept our behavior related to those beliefs, but you must appreciate our right to those beliefs. Our beliefs come from our heritage, history, conformity and the nature of the closeness of our culture. Our cultural beliefs may be subconscious and inherent.

Understand our values and respect them. Our values are geographically represented in artifacts, and, until you understand our values held in those artifacts, you will not gain our respect or trust. You must realize that the mystic symbolism in our artifacts is our connection as a group.

How do we learn—what and whom will we accept? Learning is an individual activity. As each person has an individual learning style, so do certain groups have certain learning styles. How we approach topics and methods and how we understand the role of the teacher and the meaning of the student/teacher relationship, all influence learning in the group.

What are our beliefs about the major culture or educator? To understand why we believe as we do, you must study the history of our interaction with members of the major culture. Has interaction been founded in mutual respect and trust? Just knowing our side of the history is not enough. A relationship has two parties. Be sure that you know the complete story of our relationship with the major culture. The elements of honesty and complete communication will ensure respect and trust.

What is the past history of our involvement with related topics? Attitudes are formed three ways: through past involvement with the attitude object; from past history with a familiar object; or from what others say about the object or similar object. Be sure that you know enough about us to know not only what our history has been with the topic of the educational program, but also what our history has been with similar topics, or even what we might have heard about the topic.

In addition to these five generic issues there are additional knowledge and skills necessary for educators to design and implement culturally relevant programs:

The development of culturally relevant curricula. In most schools, curricula in health education for elementary as well middle, junior high and secondary school are textbooks. If a textbook is not used, a state-approved or commercial curriculum may serve as the vehicle for the health education program. Unfortunately, many of these curricula and textbooks do not address the specific issues related to multiethnic groups. This being the case, content that is taught needs to be adapted to make it culturally relevant.

An example of a culturally relevant curriculum would be content taught that is specifically related to the multiethnic groups represented in the classroom. Such issues as specific health problems, health care, cultural values and religious practices that affect health should be considered and included. Content taught should include information directly related to environmental factors and living conditions, behavior, health risks, genetics and other factors which influence the health of multiethnic learners. This serves two purposes: (1) multiethnic students can relate and contribute to the discussion, and (2) a multicultural approach helps others develop an appreciation of cultures other than their own. Fortunately, health education lends itself to understanding cultural differences since it is behavior oriented. It is also based on individual beliefs, knowledge and values derived from one's culture, and these, in turn, reflect health behaviors of the culture. As a result, health education is a natural subject to teach from a cultural point of view.

Choosing effective classroom instructional teaching methods and strategies is just as important as developing culturally relevant curricula. It is important to know the student's background when designing ways for teaching health. There are two major factors that should be taken into consideration in developing methods and teaching strategies relevant to multiethnic groups. First, it is necessary to understand how individuals from different cultures learn best. Second, it is important to understand the determinants which could encourage or impede the student's participation in the learning process.

The following examples cited by Baruth and Manning (1992) are an attempt to explain how learning styles and cultural determinants could influence multiethnic learners:

- Asian learners seldom reveal their opinions or their abilities voluntarily, or dare to challenge their teachers. Even when they know an answer to a teacher's question, they may choose to sit quietly—as though they do not know. Expecting Asian learners to participate in discussion may jeopardize their families' name or reputation. Reprimanding Asian learners in front of peers or writing their names on the board may be far more damaging to the Asian child than to the Anglo child.

- According to Hale and Benson (cited in Baruth and Manning, 1992), African-American people tend to prefer focusing on people and their activities rather than things. Group activities, storytelling and cooperative learning would be helpful learning strategies for African-American learners. They also have a sensitivity to nonverbal clues and are well-developed in verbal and motor skills. Providing African Americans too many worksheets and drill times would defeat the learning process.

- Cultural characteristics of the Hispanic learner that should be taken into consideration when designing learning activities include not wanting to be set apart, even for excellence. Thus, the teacher should set aside opportunities for group work where the group will excel, not the individual. "Machismo" plays a significant role in the Puerto Rican culture and influences the behavior and attitudes of adolescent males. This relates to manhood, the courage to fight, keeping one's word and protecting one's name. Teaching strategies that provide opportunities for "machismo" to be exercised would satisfy sociocultural needs while at the same time fostering a positive learning environment.

- Native American cultural characteristics that influence learning include speaking softer to make a point, a carefree spirit, being unconcerned with time, expecting few rules, learning through legends, patience and a passive temperament. The teacher of health education would be wise to consider these characteristics when deciding how health content should be taught to Native-American learners. Learning activities that involve storytelling and limited verbal interaction would be appropriate.

Communication techniques can influence the teacher's ability to relate to and teach multiethnic students. "Communication not only involves what you say and how you say it, but also what you imply and what your listener perceives. Education can be effective only if the teacher and the student perceive the communication process to be positive and profitable" (Frazee and Johnson, 1993). One's teaching style represents his or her personality which in turn reflects the way he or she communicates with students. Communication is a two-way process: giving and receiving. Therefore, when communicating to students, the teacher must not only be effective in terms of oral communication but also in the art of listening. This is especially true when a student speaks broken English and is difficult to understand. This can be frustrating to both the teacher and the student and calls for patience. Sensitivity to the student's inability to communicate in English is the first prerequisite to listening and understanding what the student is trying to communicate.

Encouragement and positive reinforcement should be offered to the students so some degree of success can be experienced, which, in turn, will help build self-confidence. In some cultures, such as Asian-American, students have been taught to listen more than speak. Not volunteering to answer questions may seem to indicate indifference. Realizing this is common of Asian Americans helps the teacher understand the reason the students seem disinterested (Baruth and Manning, 1992). Some teachers "may view silence as awkward or wasteful of time. However, some cultures are quite comfortable with periods of silence. Conversely, some cultures consider it entirely appropriate to speak before the other person has finished talking..." (Frazee and Johnson, 1993). Distance between speakers is also a factor in the communication process. North Americans generally prefer a distance of thirty inches between each other, while Arabs are comfortable at eight inches (Lobenthal, cited in Pine and Hilliard, 1989). Some cultures also communicate with a great deal of emotional expression. Therefore, when communicating they may express joy or happiness more openly than Anglo Americans.

Not only is it important for educators to be able to communicate effectively with students but also to communicate and relate to parents. Educators can easily intimidate parents by the way they speak, act and look. For a parent of a different culture, intimidation may be a major factor in inhibiting a positive relationship. Treating parents with respect and courtesy, along with patience and recognition of cultural differences, provides a positive atmosphere for effective communication. The specific techniques important in communicating with parents are the same as with students. Showing interest in the customs and cultural heritage of parents will do wonders in establishing effective relationships.

Unfortunately, parents of minority children may not volunteer to meet with teachers or school authorities unless a crisis arises. This may be due to the discomfort they experience because they are intimidated by the teacher. A major effort should be made to help parents develop a comfort level with their children's schools and teachers.

Last, but not least, educators must be aware of their own biases toward multiethnic groups. Sometimes the bias is blatant and known by the individual as well as others. In other instances, a bias might be subliminal and the individual may not be aware of her or his prejudice. In this case, educators need to be helped by others so they will realize their bias and can take steps to change. Individual and group exercises during preservice as well as inservice education can assist teachers and administrators in identifying their biases toward people of different ethnic backgrounds.

The Role of Universities in Preparing Culturally Sensitive Teachers of Health Education

As mentioned earlier, teacher education programs must address the issue of multiethnic classrooms as well as subject content when preparing teachers in order to be accredited. There are different ways in which prospective teachers can be introduced to teaching in multiethnic classrooms. The first is through integration of multiethnic education in courses offered by colleges of education. Courses such as psychology of learning, sociology of education, educational media and technology, teaching methods, foundations of education, and growth and development should address the issues involved when teaching diverse populations. In addition, many colleges of education can provide opportunities for students, during their student teaching experience, to work with culturally diverse students.

A second approach in preparing teachers of health education to teach in multiethnic classrooms is to integrate the knowledge and skills regarding multicultural education into courses required in health education. An example of this would be including socio-economic, religious and culturally specific information as it pertains to populations who have specific health problems. This information could be addressed in courses on alcohol and drug education, human sexuality and family life, communicable and chronic diseases, and curriculum and methods, to name a few. By integrating cultural differences in health education courses, the future teacher of health education will have a better understanding of the health status and practices of multiethnic groups.

A third approach in teacher preparation would be a specific course on multiethnic or multicultural education. This could be offered by a college of education or perhaps a health education department. Pahnos (1992), suggests that departments of health education in colleges and universities must include multicultural education throughout teacher preparation programs. However, just one preservice course on multicultural education, or, more specifically, health education, may not adequately address the issue. Therefore, diversity should be inherent in every syllabus and course outline throughout the entire undergraduate program.

A fourth approach in preparing health education teachers in multiethnic education is through a variety of seminars, workshops or special programs offered by the health education department or university. Departments could invite teachers who have had experience teaching in multiethnic classrooms. Inviting special guests to campus who have had experience in working with diverse groups can be extremely helpful to prospective health educators. These individuals have credibility and can approach the topic of multiethnic health education in a realistic way.

In addition to guest speakers, health education majors and minors should be encouraged to attend university events which focus on the history, culture and current issues regarding racism, prejudice and multiculturalism. Many campuses have designated special programs for the purpose of better understanding different cultures. Students should be encouraged to attend these in order to develop an understanding of different cultures.

In addition, general education or university program courses may be offered that relate to specific cultures such as Black history or Latin American studies. Health education majors and minors who desire to teach in schools of diverse cultures are encouraged to take these courses as university requirements or as electives. Finally, future health education teachers, who know they will be teaching in schools where English is spoken as a second language, should develop proficiency in a foreign language.

Inservice Training for Cultural Literacy

Several teachers have never had an opportunity to develop multiethnic teaching skills. Therefore it is imperative that inservice programs be conducted so teachers can become aware of how they can have a greater impact on culturally diverse learners. Nicholai-Mays and Davis (1986), have designed a model for teacher inservice programs in multicultural urban schools. The authors list six goals of the inservice program along with activities that would foster the accomplishment of each goal.

1. The program would assist teachers to choose effective classroom instructional methods. Introduction to teaching methods such as the use of learning centers, cooperative learning, team teaching, peer tutoring, mastery learning and the laboratory approach, along with roleplaying and effective questioning techniques, would be covered.

2. The program would assist teachers in curriculum matters. This would include inviting speakers who are knowledgeable about evaluating and developing curriculum materials used in multiethnic classrooms. These individuals possibly might be provided by the state education agency, university faculty or experienced classroom teachers.

3. The program would assist teachers in improving their self-awareness, empathy and positive interpersonal relationships within the classroom. Activities in achieving this would be small group experiences where values clarification, sensitivity training and listening skills could be practiced.

4. The program would assist teachers in classroom management and use of discipline techniques. This goal should be specifically designed in addressing behavioral problems of individuals of diverse cultures. Most important would be an understanding of the reasons undesirable behaviors exist and techniques in altering these behaviors.

5. The program will assist teachers to relate more positively to parents and more effectively involve them in school affairs. The main purpose of this goal is to maximize good school/home relations. Skills and techniques for improving communication in conferencing with parents representing multiethnic groups, possible extracurricular activities planned for both parents and children and involvement of parents working as volunteers in the classroom and as resource speakers in the school could be explored.

6. The program will assist teachers to develop a greater cultural awareness. Activities to reach this goal could include workshops, guest speakers, field trips and simulations. A variety of specific topics could be addressed such as cultural pluralism, racism, positive contributions of minorities, nonverbal communication, learning styles, stereotypes and myths about ethnic groups.

In addition to the above-mentioned goals, health education teachers should be given the opportunity to understand cultures as they relate to the various health issues. This would include those factors already addressed in this chapter.

Groups Responsible for Inservice Training

The responsibility for inservice training can be assumed by four basic groups. One of these groups includes professional associations in health education such as the American School Health Association or Association for the Advancement of Health Education, which has provided a number of workshops on cultural diversity in health education. Other health education professional associations have addressed the topic at their annual conferences and in special workshops. Professional associations can also prepare publications which address the issues of teaching health education to multiethnic groups. Included would be curricula, teaching strategies and reports on the health status of minority groups.

Universities can also play a role in providing inservice training for classroom teachers of health education. Departments of health education can offer graduate courses in teaching multiethnic health education or provide seminars, workshops and inservice training on an individual or group basis to classroom teachers. Furthermore, faculty in departments of health education with an expertise in teaching multiethnic groups can serve as consultants to teachers. This could include conducting a class and demonstrating various teaching techniques. Universities, as well as professional associations, could also develop media, such as video tapes and interactive videos, to assist teachers in becoming more proficient in addressing multicultural issues or developing teaching skills for working with diverse populations.

A third group responsible for inservice would be local education authorities, who could provide inservice training for all teachers on the topic of multiethnic education. Public schools should allow teachers professional development days to attend conferences, seminars, workshops or courses that would assist them in being more effective health educators with multiethnic groups.

Public schools could also develop a mentor system where a teacher who has a proven track record of successful teaching with multiethnic groups could assist other teachers. This could involve team teaching, demonstrations, consultation or observation in the classroom.

Teacher associations or unions could serve as the fourth group to deliver inservice training. This could be done at the local or state level during meetings or conferences or in cooperation with the local education authority, as an inservice program. Teacher associations and unions have access to experts on the topic of multiethnic education, and through their organizational structure they can provide inservice programs.

Self study is a final means of inservice. This could be done by using printed materials as well as electronic media developed and marketed by commercial companies or professional associations. This would include books, curricula, special reports and papers, audio recordings as well as videos. Published literature and educational media can be extremely helpful to the health educator who is interested in learning how to be more effective in teaching health education to multiethnic groups. Additional means of self study are mentioned by Baruth and Manning (1992), who suggest ways teachers can attempt to better understand the culturally diverse learner:

- Read books and journal articles on cultural diversity related to teaching and learning.
- Request information from organizations and government agencies.
- Meet with culturally diverse learners and their families to understand what it means to be culturally different.
- When attending conferences, take advantage of programs on cultural diversity. Attend conferences that focus on teaching multiethnic learners.

- Read books and magazines that are written primarily for children and adolescents.

Conclusion

The health educator in today's schools must have expertise and confidence in teaching health education to a variety of multiethnic groups. It is unethical and a disservice to teach health education to multiethnic learners from an Anglo-American, middle-class perspective. Recognizing cultural differences is the first step in becoming an effective health educator. We must, by all means, have a sensitivity to different cultures, which includes a knowledge of the language, religion, values and beliefs, access to health care and health status of multiethnic groups that attend public schools. Preservice as well as inservice education must address the issues of teaching diverse cultures. This can be done in a variety of ways by professional preparation programs, associations, unions or commercial enterprises.

Teachers of health education have opportunities to capitalize on cultural differences that affect one's health. The subject matter is natural, due to the fact that the health of individuals can be influenced by their values and beliefs. These, in turn, reflect their culture. The health educator who is cognizant of this will be more successful in meeting the individual needs of his or her students.

References

Baruth, L. G., and M. L. Manning. 1992. *Multi-cultural education of children and adolescents.* Needham Heights, MA: Allyn and Bacon.

Centers for Disease Control and Prevention. 1992. The changing face of America: Reweaving the tapestry of America. Visual materials.

Corner, T. 1984. *Education in multicultural societies.* New York: St. Martins Press.

Davidman, R. 1990. Multi-cultural teacher education and supervision: A new approach to professional development. *Teacher Education Quarterly* (Summer): 40.

Frazee, I., and L. Johnson. 1993. *Cultural awareness and sensitivity: A crucial component to the success of comprehensive school health education.* Reston, VA: Association for the Advancement of Health Education.

Ghazizadeh, M. 1992. Islamic health sciences: A model for health education and promotion. *Journal of Health Education* 23 (4): 227-231.

Gonzalez, U. M., J. T. Gonzalez, V. Freeman and B. Howard-Pitney. 1991. *Health promotion in diverse cultural committees.* Palo Alto, CA: Health Promotion Resource Center, Stanford Center for Research in Disease Prevention.

Heimlich, J. E., and E. Van Tilburg. 1987. Subcultures and educators—concerns of membership in education. Paper presented at the AAACE Conference, 22 October. Washington, DC.

Hunter, W. A. 1974. *Multi-cultural education through competency-based teacher education.* Washington, DC: American Association of Colleges of Teacher Education.

Leslie, M., and C. Mikanowicz. 1992. The significance of cultural differences and characteristics in program development. *Wellness Perspectives: Research, Theory and Practice* 9 (1): 24-23.

Michigan Department of Public Health. 1988. Minority health in Michigan: Closing the gap. Lansing, MI: Michigan Department of Public Health.

Nicholai-Mays, S., and J. Davis. 1986. In-service training of teachers in multicultural urban schools. A Systematic Model. *Urban Education* (July): 169-179.

Pahnos, M. 1992. The continuing challenge of multicultural health education. *The Journal of Health Education* 62 (1): 24-26.

Pine, G. J., and H. G. Hillard. 1989. *Accenting behaviors for cultural diversity: HBCD.* Pending publication.

Robinson, J., E. Ames and C. Olsen. 1991. *Guidelines of AAHE/ACATE review of health education basic level programs.* Reston, VA: Association for the Advancement of Health Education.

Standards, procedures, and policies for the accreditation of professional education units. 1992. Washington, DC: The National Council for Accreditation of Teacher Education.

Chapter 14

Preservice Education for Multicultural Understanding

Deborah A. Fortune, PhD, CHES

The face of the United States and United States schools is changing. The schools are becoming increasingly composed of students from different cultural backgrounds. Demographic projections indicate that by the year 2000 one out of every three students will be a racial/ethnic minority. In some metropolitan areas, racial/ethnic minorities already make up the majority of the school population. There are more children from single-parent households—children whose parents are not married and children of teenage mothers. One in ten families live below the poverty line. Approximately 14 percent of school-age children do not speak English at home (Hodgkinson, 1989; Matiella, 1991; U.S. Census Bureau, 1992a, 1992b).

What are some of the consequences of the demographic changes and trends? More students entering schools will have the following characteristics:
- be from diverse racial/ethnic backgrounds

- be from diverse family backgrounds
- be from diverse socioeconomic backgrounds
- have limited English proficiency and language differences

Each year school districts introduce thousands of new teachers into the teaching profession. The majority are Anglo/Northern European females whose backgrounds may stand in sharp contrast to the backgrounds of the students they will teach. The question is, "Are prospective teachers prepared to teach culturally diverse classes?" The literature indicates that most new teachers, as well as veterans, have had no methodology classes and training in multicultural health education (Rodriguez, 1984; AACTE, 1980).

Prospective teachers will face the challenge of providing multicultural health education at all levels in the classroom, although many have had no or only limited training in multicultural health education. The purpose of this chapter is to provide information on teacher preparation in multicultural health education and delivery systems to prepare teachers to teach health education in the multicultural classroom.

Preservice Education Program

Multicultural understanding is fundamental to the health education of all children, not only children from racial/ethnic minority backgrounds but also those from Anglo/Northern European families. It is important for teachers to be aware of the many cultures within the classroom because this awareness provides the foundation for true multiculturalism. For teachers to recognize and appreciate the diversity of cultures in the classroom, training in multiculturalism is crucial. This section provides information on what prospective teachers in training need to know about multicultural health education and competencies. Preservice teachers need at least the following knowledge and skills related to multicultural health education.

Cognitive Competencies

Prospective teachers need to know the following (Baptiste and Baptiste, 1980; Bennett, 1990):

- Many cultures exist.
- Culture influences the decisions and behavior of students.
- Culture influences health status of students.
- Differences exist.
- Each student has a culture.
- Some contributions of different racial/ethnic groups.
- How groups of people have been treated in the United States and the consequences of the treatment.
- The cultural experience in both a contemporary and historical setting of at least two ethnic/racial or culture groups.
- Communication styles.
- Linguistic diversity.
- Learning styles of racial/ethnic minority groups.

Skills Competencies

Prospective teachers should be able to (Baptiste and Baptiste, 1980; Saville-Troike, 1978):

- Plan a multicultural program for the classroom.
- Design lessons that lead students to think critically about what they observe, hear or read related to multicultural concepts.
- Design lessons that help students break down stereotypes and promote respect for diversity.
- Select/develop teaching strategies that support the concepts of equity and express value for diversity.
- Identify stereotypes in teaching aids (e.g., textbooks, films).
- Identify values and attitudes that are part of the "hidden curriculum."

- Incorporate multicultural perspectives into all aspects of teaching.
- Encourage students' pride in their own heritage.
- Identify biases and deficiencies in existing curriculum and both commercial and teacher-prepared materials for instruction.
- Develop a model for the development and implementation of a curriculum reflective of cultural pluralism within the K through 12 school.
- Design, develop and implement an instructional module/unit using strategies and materials that will make the module/unit multicultural.

Multicultural content should be integrated throughout the curricula of preservice teacher education and health education programs. However, in many health education and education programs at the collegiate level this is not the case. At the very least, a student in preservice education should take one course in multicultural education or multicultural health education and have a practicum or field experience in a culturally diverse setting. The course should contain but not be limited to the following content areas (Saville-Troike, 1978; Bennett, 1990; Tiedt and Tiedt, 1990):

- definition of multicultural health education
- why multicultural health education is important
- demography and demographic projection
- culture and acculturation
- health problems of racial/ethnic minorities
- family
- communication styles and ethnicity
- language diversity and education
- professional capacities educators should possess
- exploring the community

- stereotypes, biases and discrimination
- tendencies and possibilities of racial/ethnic minorities
- learning styles
- multicultural health education teaching strategies
- concepts and strategies for multicultural classrooms

Delivery Systems

Multicultural health education is developmental and emergent. A variety of techniques and delivery systems are used to influence the teachers' and prospective teachers' knowledge, understanding, attitudes and skills. The techniques and delivery systems include workshops, one-day inservice training sessions, institutes of several weeks' duration, teacher education, graduate and undergraduate courses, self-instruction modules, and field-based and clinical experiences (Baptiste and Baptiste, 1980).

According to Baptiste and Baptiste (1980), most preservice education programs involved in multiculturalism can be categorized into one of three typology levels. Each of the levels of multiculturalism have readily identifiable parameters or characteristics.

Level I

This level is content oriented. It is characterized by a single culture or ethnic course—usually a survey course on a minority group. These courses might include Minority Health Issues, Health Problems of African-American Children, or Cultural Diversity in the Classroom. Level I is also characterized by workshops, seminars, conferences, ritual celebrations and holiday observations. There is generally a lack of clear-cut programmatic goals and objectives (Baptiste and Baptiste, 1980).

Probably the most obvious characteristic of Level I is its lack of institutionalization. The courses are usually not required, having an elective status. The origin of Level I is usually external pressures such as certification requirements, accreditation standards, social pressures and court decisions (Baptiste and Baptiste, 1980).

Level II

Level II is described as systematic incorporation of the content for multicultural education into the core of the teacher education program. This level is characterized by the following features: a set of interrelated courses, degree programs, certification programs, and diverse faculty and student body. Level II has a broader conceptual framework for incorporating multiculturalism into the teacher education program. There is also a theoretical referent link with practice. Specific courses and related experiences are a formalized part of the training program. The most obvious feature of this level is that a program is continuously progressing through a succession of changes toward multiculturalism (Baptiste and Baptiste, 1980).

Level III

Level III is characterized by the fact that the entire education program and its related components are permeated by a philosophical orientation of multiculturalism. Other characteristics of this level include less emphasis on isolated courses and a racially diverse faculty and student body. Ethnic and cultural diversity are not just discussed as isolated concepts but are integrated throughout the general and professional studies. The principles of recognition and respect for cultural diversity underlie instruction of the courses at this level. It is this kind of conceptual framework—embedded multiculturalism incorporated in every course and syllabus—that is recommended for the teacher preparation program (Baptiste and Baptiste, 1980).

Field Experience

"Learn by doing" has been and still is a popular paradigm in education. Therefore, the teaching experience or field practicum is probably the single most important aspect in teacher education programs. Multicultural activities and considerations should be interwoven throughout the field-based and clinical experiences. For example, how does a preservice education student reared in the suburbs become aware of the needs and complexities of children from the inner city? Field experience in a culturally diverse setting is a great opportunity to provide multicultural and multiethnic experience for preservice education students, particularly for students whose life experience has been, for the most part, monocultural.

However, field-based and clinical experiences are mostly limited to the senior year of study. In some cases, the field experience may be in a school where the culturally diverse population is limited. With creative planning and scheduling, early supervised field-based and clinical experiences with a multicultural aim can be incorporated into the preservice program. Preservice education programs need to provide field-based experience, other than the teaching practicum, in a variety of social settings in order for the students to have multicultural experiences (Kohut, 1980).

According to Kohut (1980), some of the ways some institutions have improved their multicultural education efforts for preservice education students included having them participate in the following field-based and clinical experiences:

- volunteer work at daycare, preschool or Head Start centers
- social interactions with racial/ethnic minorities
- volunteer work at short- and long-term juvenile detention centers and halfway houses, providing services such as tutoring
- interactions with senior citizens by volunteering at community centers, hospitals and long-term health care facilities

- involvement in youth-oriented programs such as Talent Search, Upward Bound, YMCA, YWCA, police athletic leagues, Boy Scouts and Girl Scouts
- involvement in school-, community- or university-sponsored drug, alcohol and related counseling clinics, and in sheltered workshops for the mentally and/or physically retarded or handicapped
- involvement in community-supported cultural and crafts fairs and shows, storefront schools and other compensatory programs sponsored by public and private funding sources
- campus activities that feature ethnic themes or foreign language or foreign cultural projects
- involvement in human and social services agencies and programs (Kohut, 1980, p. 79)

To enhance the student teaching practicum in terms of multicultural experience, the following recommendations were made by Kohut (1980):

- Provide opportunities for student teaching practicums in urban, suburban and rural settings.
- Provide pre-student and post-student teaching workshops and courses to prepare student teachers to deal with "culture shock" or cultural differences.
- Provide opportunities of a wide and diverse nature for student teachers.
- Involve all qualified faculty in the college or school of education in supervising student and intern teachers. (Kohut, 1980, p. 88-89)

Conclusion

Multicultural health education is a relatively new curriculum consideration for preservice education. Efforts have been made to deal with issues related to multicultural education in general. However, much still needs to be done in the area of multicultural health education. The following are three areas of recommendations.

Reform teacher preparation programs. With schools becoming more culturally diverse, prospective teachers need to be professionally trained and prepared to deal with diversity in the classrooms.

- Multicultural health education needs to permeate the curriculum.
- Preservice education students need at least one course in multicultural health education.
- Preservice education students should have field-based and clinical experiences in culturally diverse settings or multiracial schools.
- Multicultural health education courses should be required courses for preservice education students.

Reform the schools.
- Public schools need to have state-mandated inclusion of multicultural health education in K-12 classrooms.
- Eliminate biases from instruction and instructional materials.
- Create bias-free classrooms.

Reform faculty preparation and training.
- Faculty in preservice education program should have professional training and competencies in preparing prospective teachers to work effectively with children from culturally diverse backgrounds.

- When possible, include faculty from different cultural backgrounds.
- Faculty members with expertise in multicultural health education should serve as resource personnel for schools in the area served by the institution.
- Institutions of higher education should encourage preservice education faculty members to develop, research and implement innovations in multicultural health education (Lezotte, 1993).

Reforming teacher preparation programs, public schools and faculty preparation presents obstacles that may impede the inclusion of multicultural health education in preservice education programs. However, once the existence of these problems is acknowledged, they can be addressed and solutions found. Multicultural health education can be a reality.

References

American Association of Colleges for Teacher Education. 1980. *Multicultural teacher education: Case studies of thirteen programs*, Vol. II. Washington, DC.

Baptiste, M. L., and H. P. Baptiste, Jr. 1980. Competencies toward multiculturalism. In *Multicultural teacher education: Preparing educators to provide educational equity*, Vol. I, ed., H. P. Baptiste, Jr., M. L. Baptiste and D. M. Gollnick, 44-72. Washington, DC: American Association of Colleges for Teacher Education.

Bennett, C. I. 1990. *Comprehensive multicultural education: Theory and practice.* Boston: Allyn and Bacon.

Hodgkinson, H. L. 1989. *The same client: The demographics of education and service delivery systems.* Washington, DC: Institute for Educational Leadership, Inc.

Kohut, S., Jr. 1980. Field experience in preservice professional studies. In *Multicultural teacher education: Preparing educators to provide educational equity*, Vol. I, ed. H. P. Baptiste, Jr., M. L. Baptiste and D. M. Gollnick, 73-93. Washington, DC: American Association of Colleges for Teacher Education.

Lezotte, L. W. 1993. Effective schools: A framework for increasing student achievement. In *Multicultural education: Issues and perspectives*, ed., J. A. Banks and C. A. Banks, 303-315. Boston: Allyn and Bacon.

Matiella, A. C. 1991. *Positively different: Creating a bias-free environment for young children.* Santa Cruz, CA: ETR Associates.

Rodriguez, F. 1984. Multicultural teacher education: Interpretation, pitfalls and commitments. *Journal of Teacher Education* 35 (2): 47-50.

Saville-Troike, M. 1978. *A guide to culture in the classroom.* Rosslyn, VA: InterAmerica Research Associates, Inc.

Tiedt, P. L., and I. M. Tiedt. 1990. *Multicultural teaching: A handbook of activities, information and resources.* Boston: Allyn and Bacon.

U.S. Census Bureau. 1992a. *1990 Census of the population: General population characteristics.* Washington, DC: U.S. Department of Commerce.

U.S. Census Bureau. 1992b. *1990 Census of the population and housing: Summary social, economic and housing characteristics.* Washington, DC: U.S. Department of Commerce.

Chapter 15

Inservice Training: The Health Teacher as Professional Learner

Veronica M. Acosta-Deprez, PhD, CHES

A s health educators, we need to prepare ourselves and our students to live and work in a culturally pluralist world. Our task is characterized by complexity and difficulty, yet it is important and valuable. We have an obligation to help our students learn to live, work and interact in this diverse society and in the global community. Therefore, we must accept the multicultural teaching challenge. We can begin by becoming aware of and participating in the countless opportunities provided by inservice professional enhancement programs and activities that deal with cultural awareness, sensitivity and training.

Defining Inservice for Health Educators

"Inservice" as a term has been used frequently in various ways and situations. Webster's dictionary (1989) defines *inservice* as "going on or continuing while one is fully employed." Other meanings include some type of help, assistance, support, commission, maintenance, repair or utility. From a teaching standpoint, inservice is synonymous with continuing education, personal enrichment and professional development for staff and teachers. The way inservice is defined determines what is undertaken in its labeling. In this chapter, the definition of inservice will include *those activities that are designed to assist individuals in planning and carrying out designated professional purposes and objectives successfully and more efficiently during their practice.*

One must consider that although a suitable definition is in place for inservice, much flexibility and dynamism should be exercised in its interpretation. In its broadest sense, inservice also includes activities that are personal rather than professional in nature (but which have some influence on the professional side) as well as activities which may not be part of professional practice but of daily living. Due to the multidimensional nature and scholarship of the area of multiculturalism, inservice activities for health teachers may include external formal professional training activities and sessions as well as internal informal personal endeavors and commitments.

It is my intent in this chapter to provide teachers with an awareness of the types of inservice programs and activities, both personal and professional, that they could participate in or develop to acquire a health education perspective based on the integration of multicultural tenets into everyday teaching. The first section provides an overview of the need for inservice activities for health educators. A suggested scope and content of inservice programs will be proposed in the next section. Then some of the main issues relating to inservice training will be explored.

Why the Need for Inservice?

There are several reasons why teachers should take part in inservice programs. A rationale is provided here, as the benefits of inservice in the general areas of teaching, health education and multicultural education are explored.

Teaching

When it comes to their work situation, sense of competence, and social status, teachers are often put at a disadvantage. Van der Wolf and Ramaekers (1991) report three main cultural themes described by Hargreaves (1980) that generally describe the teaching experience:

1. The level of professional status of teaching is low.
2. The sense of competence of school teachers is low since it is less based on systematic knowledge than other professions.
3. Teaching is a profession where the practitioner usually works in solitude.

Teachers work alone in the classroom. They spend little time in pedagogic discourse and consultation with other teachers. It is a "profession in which one has to teach oneself. Beginning teachers often receive no help from experienced colleagues which often leads to an intuitive approach..." (van der Wolf and Ramaekers, 1991).

Due to the solitary nature of teaching, inservice programs emerge as an essential tool in augmenting the teaching potential. Numerous benefits of inservice programs have been well documented in educational literature. For example, a few studies have shown that teachers' participation in inservice programs has resulted in more positive teaching attitudes and renewed enthusiasm for their subject and field (Shapiro, 1981; Gaff, 1992). Inservice activities also provide teachers with a sense of competence and security in their work, promote greater social contact between colleagues as well as participation in the larger society, and provide a venue for mutual professional dialogue (Thelen, 1973).

Health Education

In additional to those mentioned above, there are several other reasons why health teachers should participate in inservice activities:

1. Health is a dynamic and ever-changing field. We are constantly besieged with new health information, reports, research, concepts, methodologies and ideologies, which result in the formation of new knowledge, attitudes and values as well as behavioral changes. Inservice activities enable teachers to stay current with new information and technology.

2. Health education is a fairly new field. Constant professional interaction and dialogue help redefine, refine and analyze the underlying conceptual structures that make up the area of health education. Inservice training provides a venue for these types of dialogue and mutual exchange.

3. Health education is aimed at improving the health status of all students. Understanding the cultural foundations upon which students' knowledge, attitudes, values and beliefs are based will enable teachers to provide health information and guidance consistent with their students' needs. Inservice workshops help teachers become aware of the various social, economic, political, ethnic and cultural factors that influence the health status of diverse populations.

4. In a study that examined the impact of inservice workshops on health teaching, Chen et al. (1990) found that inservice training significantly improved teachers' perceived competencies in health education and raised their comfort level and prepared-

ness in teaching health. A similar study by Acosta-Deprez (1992) involving multicultural health education exhibited comparable results.

5. Kingery et al. (1991) conducted a summer institute for health teachers in a research setting where teachers came in direct contact with current leaders in health research and health education methodologies. The institute brought about favorable outcomes for teachers, particularly by helping them build their own sense of empowerment over new health research information. Health research information which was otherwise incomprehensible was transferred to them in ways that were practical and immediately applicable in the classroom setting.

Multicultural Health Education

Inservice may be, to a large extent, the sole means through which teaching competencies that relate to multicultural health education are acquired. In a study investigating teachers' perceived competencies on multicultural health education, Acosta-Deprez and Monroe (1993) found that prospective teachers perceived their teacher preparation programs to be inadequate in terms of preparing them to teach multicultural health education.

Strategies for requiring a multicultural education course, or placing emphasis on multicultural learning environments have been the target of many teacher preparation programs; however, implementation has been fragmented, weak or has not been regarded with highest priority as yet (Levine and Cureton, 1992). Although multiculturalism is becoming widespread throughout higher education, Levine and Cureton (1992) state that, "...the change has not been systematic...some institutions have been more affected than others." Furthermore, the change has seldom been comprehensive.

Inservice programs provide a venue in which personal, social and professional interaction takes place. The attainment of a multicultural education perspective may be futile without such interaction as, according to Gaff (1992), "The idea of learning is to transcend personal experience and develop wisdom based on the experience of others." Gaff reiterates the need for faculty development programs which encourage "difficult dialogues" in which people examine their own views and emotional roots and where the risk of sharing deeply held beliefs is commonplace, because these activities touch the very roots of multicultural learning.

Participation in inservice activities facilitates engagement in more personal, interactive, reflective, experiential and collaborative methods of teaching and learning—all of which makes the multicultural education field unique among other areas of instruction.

The following section discusses the scope and content of an inservice program that specifically addresses multicultural health education strategies.

Scope and Content of Inservice Programs on Multicultural Health Education

To propose an inservice program that would cover all aspects of multicultural health education is impossible. The scope and content of multicultural health education programs will vary according to the differing needs and situations of each audience. There are several approaches to defining the scope and sequence of an inservice professional enhancement program for health educators. In this section, I would like to propose and explore two approaches which could be used as guides by health educators in seeking or developing inservice programs that enrich their professional competencies in working with multicultural environments. These approaches are the Multicultural Health Education Area Responsibilities Approach and the Multicultural Comprehensive School Health Education Approach.

Multicultural Health Education Area Responsibilities Approach

The Multicultural Health Education Area Responsibilities Approach bases its scope and content on the general Area Responsibilities and Competencies for Health Educators as designated by the National Commission for Health Education Credentialing, Inc. (Rubinson and Alles, 1984). In this approach, multicultural elements are integrated into the seven general area responsibilities. Some questions are posed relative to general competencies under each area. The object here is for health educators to ask themselves whether they exhibit the skills necessary to carry out their tasks as health educators and if they are able to perform these functions within culturally diverse classrooms and communities.

Responsibilities

1. Assess individual and community needs for multicultural health education.
   - What specific health practices, beliefs, values, attitudes and habits do I need to become aware of in order to facilitate assessment of the health needs of a particular group or community? What factors have influenced the existence and/or occurrence of these needs?
   - What general as well as specific cultural traits or characteristics do members of the community portray that enable me to understand, appreciate and empathize with their health status and needs?
   - What data and resources are available about specific groups

that describe their social and cultural environments, growth and developmental factors/patterns, and interests?

- What approaches may be utilized for mutual, effective and interactive communication to take place between the program developers and workers and the community members?
- What are those health needs that require the expertise of health professionals or nonhealth professionals? What are the needs that require professional or nonprofessional assistance?
- What types of resources are needed in order to plan health education programs that are consistent with the needs and culture of a particular community?

2. Plan effective multicultural health education programs.
   - What skills, proficiencies, expertise and abilities do I need to be able to plan multicultural health education objectives and programs?
   - Which community organizations, resource people and potential community participants could be called upon to provide assistance in program planning?
   - Which health needs should take precedence over others when addressing priorities?
   - What would the scope and sequence of a multicultural health education program consist of, given the culture of the community with which I will be working?
   - What program objectives should be designed that are sensitive to and consistent with the values, attitudes, beliefs and practices of the members of the community?

3. Exhibit competence in carrying out planned multicultural health education programs.

- What characteristics, abilities, expertise, skills and proficiencies are needed to exhibit competence in carrying out planned multicultural health education objectives?
- What culturally appropriate and socially sensitive types of instructional materials are available that will enable me to carry out multicultural health education objectives effectively?
- What resource organizations, agencies, learning centers and bureaus are available that may assist and support me in the planning and implementation of health programs for multicultural populations?
- What methods and media should I be aware of that may be best suited to implement the program for specific learners? What teaching methods are preferred and learning styles exhibited by particular groups of learners? What materials are available that may help me learn and apply these in my program?

4. Evaluate effectiveness of multicultural health education programs.
   - What evaluation measures could be used to measure the accomplishment of program objectives? Which measures are nonbiased and nonpartial?
   - What specific types of quantitative as well as qualitative evaluation measures are prescribed in measuring program objectives relative to particular groups?
   - What competencies do health educators need to be able to interpret evaluation results more effectively?
   - Which activities have been effective in facilitating desired outcomes? Which have not?
   - In what ways could nonsubjective, nonbiased feedback be provided to the learners?

5. Coordinate the provision of multicultural health education services.
   - What skills and competencies are needed to be able to coordinate health education services that address the needs of multicultural populations?
   - How can cooperation among program personnel be facilitated?
   - What health agencies and organizations exist that are responsive to the needs of multicultural groups? In what ways can their collaboration be fostered in relation to program planning?
   - What competencies are needed in order to be able to organize multicultural health education inservice programs for teachers, volunteers and other interested personnel?

6. Act as a resource person in multicultural health education.
   - What information, skills, competencies, expertise and experiences are needed in order to act as a resource person for multicultural health education?
   - What competencies, skills, expertise, experiences are needed in order to be of help to those who request assistance in solving health problems of specific population groups?
   - Am I able to carefully interpret and respond to requests for health information on specific populations and cultural groups?
   - What skills are needed in order to select and disseminate health education materials catering to specific groups?

7. Communicate health education needs, concerns and resources of different gender, social, economic, ethnic, exceptionally different and cultural groups.

- What personal characteristics, skills, experiences and competencies are needed in order to have the ability to interpret concepts, purposes and theories of multicultural health education?
- What societal value systems impact on the effectiveness of health education programs?
- What culturally appropriate methods and techniques of communication are available in disseminating health information?
- What approaches may be utilized in fostering cooperation, collaboration and communication between health care professionals and their culturally diverse consumers?

Multicultural Comprehensive School Health Education Approach

Teachers who are a part of a comprehensive school health program will benefit from inservice programs that focus on strengthening their practice as well as on enabling them to carry out their roles in working with culturally diverse learners.

A comprehensive school health program is an "organized set of policies, procedures and activities designed to protect and promote the health and well-being of students and staff" (Meeks and Heit, 1992). Within a comprehensive school health program, the health teacher, as part of the school health advisory committee, takes part in three major roles: school health education, creating a healthy school environment and providing school health services.

To address the needs of diverse learners, multicultural principles must be integrated into each of the above-mentioned roles. A perspective of multiculturalism is provided here in light of the health educator's three roles within a comprehensive school health education program.

School Health Education

School health education is the "component of the comprehensive school health program which includes the development, delivery and evaluation of a planned instructional program and other activities for students in preschool through grade 12, for parents and for school staff, and is designed to influence positively the health knowledge, attitudes and skills of individuals" (Meeks and Heit, 1992).

Teachers attempting to participate in school health education for culturally diverse groups of students may benefit from inservice programs that cover the following three teacher competencies (Hunter, 1974):

Competency I—Understanding Human Growth and Development. Teachers must recognize that each individual is worthwhile and unique and that their behaviors are caused and not arbitrary. Teachers must be aware that each individual has dignity and integrity and wants to achieve success. The principles of human growth and development may not be generalized to everyone, but when these concepts are applied, teachers need to understand the possible results. It is equally important to understand that the development of social relationships differs among students and that teachers may need to provide the venue through which these relationships are fostered and enhanced. As the environment plays a role in influencing learning outcomes and abilities, teachers should be able to create an environment conducive to learning.

Competency II—Planning and Preparing for Instruction. Learners exhibit a wide range of interests and achievement levels, value systems and standards, cultural backgrounds and language patterns. In order to effectively accomplish instructional objectives, a variety of instructional approaches consistent with these learning backgrounds must be planned. Hence, the acquisition of knowledge about these instructional approaches, particularly those that have been proven to be effective in reinforcing the learning abilities of particular cultural groups is essential. Teachers need to engage learners in nontraditional modes of learning that require inquiry, creativity, sensitivity, conceptualization, critical and analytical thinking, rational decision making, and knowledge of cause and effect rather than the "business as usual" approaches. Instructional activities that bring about the best outcomes in their learners have to be utilized.

Competency III—Performing Instructional Functions. Effective teaching for multicultural populations begins with the teacher's ability to demonstrate appropriate written and oral communication skills. Learning to speak the language of learners will be very valuable. Teachers should be able to adjust instruction to the context, content, individual learning styles, modes and rates of growth of the learners. Instructional materials, procedures and activities should be analyzed in terms of cultural appropriateness. When unexpected events or disruptive activities occur, teachers should be able to manage these as well as handle strong feelings and interruptions in class. In addition, teachers need to exhibit reassuring, reinforcing and supportive traits towards all the responses of their learners.

School Health Environment

Healthful school environment is that division of a comprehensive school health program that "focuses on the school day, school building and surrounding area, and specific school activities, procedures and policies that protect the health and safety of faculty, staff and students" (Meeks and Heit, 1992).

Health teachers' duties are not confined merely to instruction but also to the promotion of an environment that is healthful and conducive to learning. This environment includes the physical, mental, spiritual and social climates within the classroom and school. An environment conducive to multicultural learning promotes characteristics of acceptance, openness and tolerance for differences. Teachers need to create both overt (as in decorating the classroom and school grounds with pictures representative of various ethnic and cultural groups) as well as covert (as in exemplifying role-model traits of being nonjudgmental, nonbiased, open and accepting of differences) ways of promoting characteristics of openness and acceptance among their students.

School Health Services

School health services is that "section of the comprehensive school health program provided by physicians, nurses, dentists, health educators and allied health personnel to appraise, protect and promote the health of students and health personnel" (Meeks and Heit, 1992).

The major role of the health teacher in school health services is the observation of physiological, attitudinal and behavioral changes that may occur among students and referral to appropriate sources for various health needs. Teachers should be aware of the health habits and behavioral patterns of students from different ethnic, religious or cultural groups in the classroom. Teachers also have to be cognizant of the health histories of their students and monitor those who may be in need of help and attention both in and outside the classroom. Various health as well as nonhealth problems may be existent among students. It would be advantageous for teachers to know the different sets of problems that students experience so as to be able to provide assistance, supervision and referral as necessary.

Several inservice programs may focus on one instead of all content areas or responsibilities. In this regard, a great deal of flexibility must be employed in considering these propositions;

one program may not necessarily cover everything in the above-mentioned scope and content approaches. Teachers need to be attentive and cognizant of programs and activities that include most of the content in each approach. Additionally, teachers should also participate in inservice programs that focus on content areas and strategies that are personally meaningful to them, as these are likewise professionally enhancing.

Issues in Inservice Training

The attainment of a multicultural perspective is a complex and ongoing process. There are many issues one may encounter in doing multicultural health education. Some are personal; others are more administrative and curricular in orientation. The kinds of issues related to inservice training for multicultural health education are very similar to those which are experienced in acquiring a multicultural perspective.

First let's examine the personal philosophical issues that pose barriers to the multicultural challenge. For numerous reasons, many teachers have preexisting notions that workshops dealing with cultural awareness or cultural diversity are solely intended for certain racial or ethnic groups, or are breeding grounds for political, cultural or social debates on controversial issues. Such is not the case. Multiculturalism, according to Gaff (1992), is a radically multidimensional rather than a unitary construct. It may mean many things to many individuals. It may include topics on gender differences, racial issues, cultural diversity, Western and non-Western cultures, international issues, sexual preference, exceptionality, class differences and physical dissimilarities. Agreement and clarity of the multicultural concept has not been reached, hence, the misperception that inservice programs address political ideologies rather than intellectual rationale may easily occur.

Working towards acquiring a multicultural perspective necessitates the need to first examine our own assumptions, our own feelings of superiority and security, confidence and assurance of the place that we have in our own cultures. Many people feel comfortable and secure in their own niches, and new knowledge and change will sometimes bring about resistance on their parts. Such resistance may be due to their ignorance of new scholarship, their racial and gender biases, and even their fear of what will happen when they expose themselves and their students to knowledge of cultures that have suffered historical subordination, oppression, hostility and struggle. "To bring these cultures into the classroom is to confront the ignominious as well as the glorious side of our history" (Wilkerson, 1992). Some teachers feel that they will not be able to manage or handle resistance, confrontation, conflict, anger, frustration and confusion among their students, as well as their own feelings of guilt. As Wilkerson (1992) continues, "This fear is very real...it is the 'self' that is really at stake here, the very notion of 'personal identity' around which liberal education has evolved."

When teachers recognize that gaps and inaccuracies exist within their knowledge base, they perceive this more as a challenge to their professional integrity than as a personal challenge to learn. "A new insight may also cause a revolution in the way one views the world" (Butler and Schmitz, 1992). For example, when students are taught that their culture of health is based on "science" and that there are non-science-based alternative health cultures that are equally appropriate from a particular ideological standpoint, this raises questions about their wisdom regarding "health" and "science" and challenges their assumptions about their own identity, knowledge base and culture.

Administrative and institutional limitations are also issues that teachers are confronted with in dealing with the multicultural challenge. Although opportunities for multicultural education programs and activities are supported by many institutions, implementation and reinforcement of these have not been thorough and ongoing. According to Banks (1989) the school should be viewed as a social system that consists of highly interrelated parts and variables. Attempts to implement multicultural education entail transforming all the major components and not just one variable. A teacher who integrates multicultural ways of teaching and learning into the classroom (e.g., critical thinking) may be frustrated in implementing these methodologies if other teachers within the same school do not reinforce them in their classrooms but still conform to traditional and conventional "business as usual" teaching approaches.

There also exists the ongoing issue of underrepresentation of culturally diverse teachers within the school. Teachers from various ethnic, exceptionally different, religious and cultural groups are not well represented in many school districts and communities. This restricts the number of teachers qualified to teach about certain cultural concepts. To a large extent, there is certainly a limited number of teachers with the required professional knowledge and experiential base to teach about multiculturalism. Very few faculty are capable and competent to teach courses on multiculturalism.

As teachers pursue the challenge of multicultural education, they will encounter several issues that may tend to obstruct their goals. Confronting one or more of these issues, however, must not limit attendance and participation in multicultural inservice programs. These programs may not guarantee total deliverance but they provide opportunities for engagement in reflective dialogue, the essential force in liberal pluralism, and, in the process, awareness of personal values and commitments.

Conclusion

The motivation to follow the challenge of multicultural health education must come from within us, if not from or in addition to the programs under which we have been trained. As teachers, our goal is to be able to address the health needs of all our students. By integrating the cultural beliefs and attitudes of our students into teaching health, we may be able to shed some light on the solution to problems of inequality in health status. One way in which this could be done is for practicing teachers to find opportunities for professional enhancement and renewal through inservice programs and activities.

In our attempt to implement multicultural health education, we must recognize that the success of our programs requires an intellectual rationale. There is a need for teachers to reexamine and clarify the purpose of teaching about other cultures. As Wilkerson (1992) states, "Any effort to change must be based on sound intellectual grounds. It should not be presented or conceptualized as a palliative to satisfy political interests, nor as a concession to students who need to 'feel good' in the classroom."

The attainment of a multicultural perspective entails lifelong learning and practice, and may not merely be undertaken exclusively through a series of cultural awareness workshops. A strong personal commitment towards multiculturalism becomes a necessary impetus as well as a reinforcing factor in attaining a multicultural perspective. As Eggleston (1981) states, "...effective teaching in multicultural situations is not a job that 'anyone can do'...a short course is not 'all that is needed'; such a belief devalues not only the teachers but also the courses."

Inherent in the multicultural education field is the element of continuity, because the exemplary goals that this field tries to actualize can never be fully attained in any society (Banks, 1989).

As health teachers, our goal is to help ourselves and our students develop the knowledge, attitudes and skills necessary to live healthy and productive lives and to function within our own communities as well as within the global community in which we live. In the words of Wilkerson (1992), our challenge calls for us to "think how we want our students to think and do what we ask our students to do—to continue learning."

References

Acosta-Deprez, V. 1992. *Enhancing multicultural health education competencies through a cultural awareness workshop for health educators.* Paper presented at the Alabama State Association for Health, Physical Education, Recreation and Dance Conference, Birmingham, Alabama, 20 November.

Acosta-Deprez, V., and D. Monroe. 1993. *Dealing with cultural diversity in a health education classroom: Are prospective teachers prepared?* Paper presented at the American Alliance for Health, Physical Education, Recreation and Dance Conference, Washington, DC, 25 March.

Banks, J. 1989. Multicultural education: characteristics and goals. In *Multicultural education: Issues and perspectives,* ed. J. Banks and C. McGee Banks, 2-25. Boston: Allyn and Bacon.

Butler, J., and B. Schmitz. 1992. Ethnic studies, women's studies and multiculturalism. *Change* 24 (1): 37-41.

Chen, W. et al. 1990. Impact of a continuing health education inservice program on teachers' competencies. *Health Education* 21 (6): 8-11.

Eggleston, J. 1981. Present provision in in-service training. In *Teaching in a multicultural society,* ed. M. Craft. Sussex, England: The Falmer Press.

Gaff. J. 1992. Beyond politics: The educational issues inherent in multicultural education. *Change* 24 (1): 31-35.

Hargreaves, D. 1980. The occupational culture of teachers. In *Teacher strategies: Exploration in the sociology of the school,* ed. P. Woods. London: Croom Helm.

Hunter, W. 1974. *Multicultural education through competency-based teacher education.* Washington, DC: American Association of Colleges for Teacher Education.

Kingery, P. , B. E. Pruitt, W. P. Buckner, M. Jibaja-Rusth and J. D. Holcomb. 1991. Empowering health teachers through a summer institute in a research environment. *Journal of Health Education* 22 (5): 291-296.

Levine, A., and J. Cureton. 1992. The quiet revolution: Eleven facts about multiculturalism and the curriculum. *Change* 24 (1): 25-29.

Meeks, L., and P. Heit. 1992. *Comprehensive school health education.* Blacklick, OH: Meeks Heit Publishing.

Rubinson, L. and W. Alles. 1984. *Health education: Foundations for the future.* Prospect Heights, IL: Waveland Press.

Shapiro, H. S. 1981. Implementing P.L. 94742 in the high school—a successful inservice training model. *Education* 2:47-52.

Thelen, H. 1973. A cultural approach to inservice teacher training. In *Improving inservice education,* ed. L. Rubin, 71-104. Boston: Allyn and Bacon.

van der Wolf, K., and P. Ramaekers. 1991. The development of professional competence and interaction: New goals for inservice training and staff development. In *The practitioner's power of choice,* ed. H. Letiche, J. van der Wolf and F. Plooij, 163-175. Amsterdam/Lisse: Swets and Zeitlinger B. V.

Webster's ninth new collegiate dictionary. 1989. Springfield, MA: Merriam-Webster, Inc.

Wilkerson, M. 1992. Beyond the graveyard: Engaging faculty involvement. *Change* 24 (1): 59-63.

Working Together:
Family and Community
Involvement

Chapter 16

Family Involvement in the Classroom and School Site

Maria E. Hernandez, MA, and Charlene A. Day, MPA, CHES

F amily involvement in health education is a crucial element in the intellectual, psychological, emotional and physical development of children. The family can both facilitate and enhance children's adoption of healthy behaviors. Families can appropriately serve as advocates or critics of school health programs. They can stimulate the mobilization of resources and secure community acceptance of comprehensive health education by participating in health promotion efforts that benefit their children as well as themselves.

Family involvement is particularly critical in multicultural settings where the variety of values, beliefs, attitudes, learning styles and languages makes health education a challenge. This chapter discusses some of the issues and challenges of family involvement in the multicultural classroom.

Changes in family structure and in society in general have had an impact on family involvement in education. This chapter demonstrates the particular importance of family involvement in health education in multicultural settings. It also offers suggestions about how family participation can facilitate the use of appropriate and culturally sensitive health education strategies and materials. A discussion of the barriers to family involvement in health education and strategies for overcoming these obstacles is included. Finally, a plan of action is presented for building community/school partnerships.

The Modern Family

In a nation that is becoming increasingly diverse, it seems obvious that a single definition for the traditional family is narrow and inappropriate. Yet in order to talk about family involvement we must have a clear understanding of what we mean by family, and how the family concept differs across cultures and generations.

The definition of family has changed over the last two decades, and the so-called traditional family has become less and less common. The typical "nuclear family" was and still is, in some areas, thought of as the *ideal* family form. Any deviations from this ideal are viewed as undesirable and even unwholesome. Nevertheless, even in the past, most families did not fit the nuclear ideal. "For many women confined to the roles of housewife and mother, the nuclear home was a prison. And for many henpecked men it was hardly a haven" (Elkin, 1991). Women's liberation, the sexual revolution, changing attitudes toward divorce, the introduction of television and new technologies, and other societal changes have caused a fundamental shift in the traditional boundaries of the nuclear family. Single-parent, two-parents working, blended, extended, and traditional one-parent-working and one-parent-home families are all variations of the post-modern family (Elkin, 1991).

Therefore, we need a much broader definition of family, especially in an increasingly multicultural society. Varying cultural norms related to family will force the definition of family to be broadened. The family should be defined by the individual, since we can no longer assume a general and common interpretation of the term. The San Diego Family Health Project, a multiethnic family-based health education intervention, defined "family" in the following way: "any group of one or more children and one or more adults who cohabit and share family functions such as food preparation and socialization of children" (Nader et al., 1986). Although this may be a broader definition of family than the traditional one, it limits the interpretation to include only those persons who are living together. For some, this definition may still be too narrow. The following general definition may be more appropriate: A family can be defined as two or more persons who may or may not be the mother and/or father of an individual, and who may or may not be blood relations or be living in the same dwelling, but who are important to the person and defined as family by the individual. Thus, a family, in its broadest interpretation, can be one or more persons significant to an individual.

The definition of family has been shaped by environmental factors. Many mothers now work outside the home, and a growing number of families are headed by single parents. Unemployment, poverty, homelessness and hunger are often experienced by many. These conditions place extreme stress and burdens on family life which, in turn, affect both the health of children and their readiness and capacity to learn.

A recent major change is that a greater number of children are cared for outside the home by a provider other than a family member. This is because more than 50 percent of women with children under the age of six are employed full- or part-time, making it necessary for children to be at home alone both before and/or after school. Consequently, contemporary parents spend less time with their children. These same parents are faced with the increasing challenge of protecting, guiding and instructing their children, who may be faced with health threats and other problems related to drugs, violence and sex (Elkin, 1991).

These changes make it extremely important for the school and the family to pool their efforts in the health education of children. This situation also underscores the importance of educators being culturally aware and sensitive to the many concerns and issues confronting all families, particularly those belonging to minority populations. These families may face additional difficulties and be disproportionately affected by health and other social problems.

Multicultural Family Involvement in Health Education

Research indicates that student scholastic achievement is directly related to family involvement. Additionally, research shows a strong relationship between family involvement and increases in student attendance, decreases in dropout rates, improvement of student attitudes and behavior, positive parent/child communication, and more family and community support of the school (Rich, 1988).

Besides the considerable research indicating that family involvement in education is very beneficial for children, much evidence also shows that parents, teachers and administrators all strongly favor family involvement in the schools (Chavkin, 1989). Contrary to some beliefs, minority families are no exception; they are generally very interested in becoming involved in their children's education.

In a study by Chavkin and Williams (1985), more than 3,000 parents and 4,000 educators were surveyed in the southwestern United States about attitudes and practices of family involvement.

More than one-third of the respondents in this study were either Black or Hispanic. Researchers found that minority parents expressed interest in participation in a variety of roles beyond the traditional ones of parents as school activity audiences, school supporters and home tutors. They were also interested in participating as co-learners, advocates and decision-makers. The general interest at this level of involvement manifests the need for involving multicultural families in effective and productive family/school partnerships.

Because families are intimately involved in the shaping of values, beliefs and attitudes regarding health in their children, family involvement becomes a vital element in a successful comprehensive school health education program. Schools must seek ways to collaborate in educating children and in empowering the family to make the home environment one that minimizes risk for health problems and promotes healthy lifestyles.

Until recently, we have largely ignored the importance of family involvement in health education from a multicultural perspective. It is evident, however, that the ability to focus from this multicultural standpoint has tremendous implications for our nation. The 1990 census has shown a dramatic increase in minority populations and particularly in the number of minority children, due to high fertility rates. By the year 2000, students of color will comprise between 30 and 40 percent of total school enrollment (Hodgkinson, 1985). The teaching force in this country, however, does not reflect the growing diversity of the students; in fact, it is becoming increasingly White and female (Center for Education Statistics, 1987). Socioeconomic differences between teachers and students' families amplify this contrast. These problems are compounded by a legacy of judicial, legislative and social disparities experienced by students of color, female students, and poor students and families in their interactions with school officials (Grant and Millar, 1992).

Families naturally share their values and beliefs with children. Initially, they have a powerful influence on the social, psychological, physical, emotional and spiritual development of their children. Parents and other family members are the fundamental models and the first teachers their children experience. Early on, children begin to learn and imitate actions, attitudes, beliefs and values related to health. They form habits concerning food, hygiene and exercise. They also imitate unhealthy behaviors such as smoking and alcohol and other drug use. Although children will have many teachers throughout their development, the role of the family is unique and extremely important. Therefore family participation in school health education is critical in enhancing a child's health, and, consequently, his or her ability to learn.

Family participation is particularly important in health education for a number of reasons:

- The family may be the only or primary source of health information.
- The family helps shape values, beliefs and perceptions with regard to health.
- The family may either encourage or discourage the use of health information and the seeking of health care by students (AAHE, 1992).

Cultural and Family Beliefs, Attitudes and Values

Health educators know that beliefs, attitudes and values influence health behavior, yet most intervention strategies fail to go beyond White mainstream norms. There are many cultural influences, beliefs and practices which could be applied to promote, maintain, or enhance health behavior. Nevertheless, health educators and program planners tend to focus on the barriers rather than the facilitators of positive health behavior (Orlandi, 1986).

Families vary in their ideas about education and health. There are many differences in beliefs and practices including who cares for and educates children of different ages and sexes, what the expectations are of children at different stages of development, and what kinds of competencies and behaviors are seen as normal or ideal. It is important, therefore, that classroom teachers and school administrators attempt to understand the family structure and expected responsibilities of their students. This understanding can be realistically portrayed and reflected in the classroom. This information provides essential guidance for the teacher when dealing with the child or the child's family member(s). It can also help the teacher understand the behaviors and attitudes of children and their families (AAHE, 1992).

Personal values, attitudes and beliefs are inseparably linked to ultimate choices in health behavior. Most health educators realize that simply exposing students to new ideas or practices will not automatically result in adoption, especially if these ideas conflict with their personal or family values. Conflicts in health-related values represent one of the most salient dilemmas and challenges for health education teachers. Consequently, an important technique employed by health educators is to help students sort through any conflicts in their health-related values.

Conflicts in health beliefs and practices can also arise between students from different cultural backgrounds. Teachers and administrators must realize that the values that one culture views as positive may be undesirable or threatening to another. The consumption of certain "healthy foods," for example, may be unacceptable for some people because of differing religious or cultural beliefs and practices. Furthermore, values commonly found in the United States may be inappropriate to some cultures. For example, some cultures concentrate on duration of life, whereas others place greater emphasis on the quality of life. Teachers, administrators and families must recognize the fact that values that influence health behavior vary from culture to culture. Figure 1 illustrates a number of contrasting values that may exist between the "mainstream" United States culture and other cultures.

Figure 1
Dichotomy of Values

U.S. "mainstream"	Some other cultures
Personal control over environment	Fate
Change	Tradition
Time dominates	Human interaction dominates
Human equality	Hierarchy/rank/status
Individualism/privacy	Group welfare
Self-help	Birthright/inheritance
Competition	Cooperation

Source: Association for the Advancement of Health Education. 1992. Training material. AAHE Cultural Awareness and Sensitivity Training Project.

In addition to values, beliefs and practices also vary across cultures. To effectively engage families in comprehensive health education, we must understand the various health-related beliefs and practices of the families of the students in the classroom.

We define belief as a conviction that a phenomenon or an object is real. Faith, trust and truth are words used to express or imply belief. Cultures vary in their beliefs about the cause, prevention and treatment of illness, and these beliefs influence health behavior. Some cultures closely tie religious beliefs to the state of health. For example, illness might be viewed as a punishment for sins, and good health may be seen as a gift from God. In addition, health care, whether traditional, folk or conventional medical practices, may vary according to specific cultural beliefs and practices. For example, some cultures do not practice preventive health techniques. If no acute symptoms exist, these individuals may be unwilling to seek health care; thus, preventive health practices, such as dental or eye exams and diabetes and cancer screening, are avoided or considered unnecessary. Insensitive health education curricula that emphasize the use of preventive health services or that promote radical changes in daily practices have the potential to cause conflict between children and their families. Teachers and administrators must work with both students and family members in order to develop an acceptable plan for multicultural health education and family involvement which recognizes and builds upon specific cultural beliefs and practices.

How Family Involvement Can Help

Individual and family values, beliefs and attitudes regarding health education topics such as nutrition, hygiene, sexuality, and alcohol and drug use have a significant impact on the effectiveness of the health education curriculum. The shape and content of the curriculum could be greatly influenced by family attitudes and opinions. Family beliefs and practices invariably affect students' health behaviors. Furthermore, since knowledge about what is healthy and unhealthy often influences behavior much less than beliefs and attitudes, it is undesirable to separate cognitive instruction about health from the many personal factors that affect health behavior. To avoid possible value conflicts, health educators often avoid discussions about morals and values related to the specific health education topic at hand. Because of this, health educators have been criticized for presenting amoral information and for providing only a limited number of perspectives regarding a particular health issue. Family involvement allows the family to ensure appropriate interpretation and guidance for their children regarding health beliefs and behavior. At the same time, families can provide support to the teachers regarding specific cultural issues or sensitive topics.

If educators hope to increase minority family involvement, they must adopt an attitude and willingness to learn about various cultures, to practice cultural sensitivity and to move toward a culturally integrated approach in their teaching. A familiarization with multicultural research on family involvement could be especially helpful in understanding the many issues both inhibiting and facilitating family participation in health education.

Strategies for Family Involvement
Some specific strategies for involving parents include the following (adapted from Debusk and Leslie, 1991):
- Address letters "Dear Family" rather than "Dear Parents."
- Do not schedule Mother/Daughter or Father/Son activities; instead schedule Family/Child activities at convenient times.
- Teachers and principals should keep each other informed of such events as divorce or death in the family of a student. Both teachers and principals should know, in the case of divorce, who is the custodial parent and what visiting and other rights the noncustodial parent has.
- If there is joint custody or co-parenting, find out who will come to parent/teacher conferences and receive school newsletters.
- Review the school's curriculum to make sure it portrays alternatives to the "traditional" family concept of a working father, stay-at-home mother and two children.
- Set up peer counseling and support groups for children of single parents and provide information to their parents about school and community resources and services.
- Offer before- and after-school childcare and activity programs.

When planning activities, be aware that single-income families often cannot afford additional expenses.

- Avoid negative labels such as "broken home."
- Reinforce the child's self-worth through self-esteem exercises, teaching responsibility and fostering pride in accomplishments.

Challenges to Multicultural Family Involvement

If minority parents have a high level of interest in their children's education, then why has their level of involvement been less than optimal? Although many health educators understand that family involvement is extremely important, there are still significant gaps in our knowledge of how to bring parents into the educational process more effectively (Underwood, 1986).

While some families experience barriers to involvement more often than others, obstacles to effective family involvement may occur regardless of cultural or ethnic status. We must identify and understand these barriers to family involvement in order to engage more families in the health education of their children. Some research has focused on barriers to family involvement in multiethnic populations. In a study which explored barriers to home/school collaboration by surveying 60 Black families and 29 teachers (28 Black and 1 Asian), two major barriers to involvement were found: lack of mutual understanding between teachers and families, and lack of planning on the part of teachers and school administrators (Leitch and Tangri, 1988). The authors suggest that both teachers and families must learn how to work together more effectively and how to collaborate on specific plans.

A number of other barriers to family involvement have also been cited in the literature. Generally, differences between teachers and parents in education level and socioeconomic level can have a negative impact on family involvement. The Metropolitan Life Survey of the American Teacher (Louis Harris and Associates, 1987), which surveyed more than 1,000 teachers and 2,000 parents of public school children, found that parents with less than a high school education were twice as likely to feel awkward about approaching school personnel as were parents with a college education.

Wells (1988) found that minority parents were occasionally intimidated by the staff and the institutional structure of the school. This was particularly true if earlier contacts with the schools had been negative. Chavkin (1989) comments that problems in parental involvement often occur because parents with less education and fewer mainstream social skills are reluctant to come to the school. This reluctance can be overcome if parent participation programs are structured appropriately.

Comer (1986) suggests that parents need clear mechanisms for involvement; simply inviting parents to the school is not enough. For example, the Yale Child Study Team (Comer, 1986) worked with low-income New Haven public schools and showed that family involvement improved dramatically through the creation of a meaningful parent participation program. A steering committee, or a school advisory counsel, made up of parents was created. Montalvo (1984) believes that it is up to the school to build the bridge between home and community. In his study "Make Something Happen" (a report on high school education for Hispanic Youth), he notes that, of the ten schools he visited, the ones most successful regarding family involvement were those that made extensive efforts to involve the parents.

The Minority Oral Health Improvement Program, which created multicultural materials ("Bright Smiles, Bright Futures" curriculum) for first graders, encouraged family participation in both the planning and evaluation of curricular materials. The program also incorporated family involvement activities that children could complete at home. These games, activities and family projects reinforced what the children learned in class. All of the family-oriented materials were developed for low-literacy families and were designed to be culturally sensitive and appropriate. The families expressed satisfaction with the materials, and the teachers reported increased family participation (Gold et al., 1992).

Other challenges to family involvement are related to the dramatic changes in family life that have occurred over the last two decades (Family Service America, 1987). An increase in the divorce rate, a rise in the number of single-parent homes, an increase in the number of working parent families, and an increase in the number of families below the poverty level have contributed to limited family involvement in the educational system. In the United States, these problems are often experienced to a greater degree among minority populations, and are consequently reflected in their level of family involvement. Response to changes in family structure will prove a significant challenge for educators and administrators. Teachers must continually consider the family structure of the students in their classrooms. We must remember that the traditional nuclear family may not always be represented in today's classroom.

A training curriculum on cultural sensitivity and awareness for health educators developed by the Association for the Advancement of Health Education (AAHE), suggests that teachers must be sensitive to the family situation of each student. School home notes should not be addressed to "mommy or daddy" specifically, but rather to the family of the student. Also, teachers should be aware that working parents may not be available for after-school or evening meetings, and that a more flexible schedule for parent/teacher meetings is needed (AAHE, 1992).

Curricular materials and take-home materials should include

multicultural images and a variety of family structures. For example, in the Bright Smiles, Bright Futures program (Gold et al., 1992), take-home materials incorporated images of children of multiethnic backgrounds and of multigeneration families. These materials enhanced participation levels and made families feel more comfortable in interacting with the school.

Some schools are beginning to respond to the needs of varying family structures. In a nationwide survey of nearly 500 principals of elementary and middle schools, 85 percent said they ensure the curriculum reflects a "variety of family types" rather than simply portraying the traditional family of a working father and a stay-at-home mother (Henderson, Marburger and Ooms, 1986). However, schools have a long way to go in addressing the needs of many families with other than "traditional" family structures. Less than one-third of the schools surveyed offered before- or after-school childcare. Only about half of the schools said they offer babysitting services during school functions. Henderson, Marburger and Ooms (1986) listed a number of common barriers to effective parent involvement, including:

- lack of transportation
- time constraints for both parents and teachers
- unavailable or inadequate childcare
- inflexible employer leave policies
- skeptical or negative attitudes of teachers and administrators towards parents
- lack of materials
- lack of knowledge and information about best practices
- lack of funding

Another barrier to family involvement in the education system is the lack of training for teachers and administrators about the best ways to involve low-income and minority parents effectively.

These issues underscore the need for schools to educate staff and to be flexible in their attempts to involve the families of their students.

In an article reporting findings from a community-based multicultural substance use prevention program, Orlandi (1986) noted several obstacles to family involvement. He commented that, in general, barriers such as language and low reading level surface when health interventions fail to consider sociocultural factors. Those who seek to foster family involvement in health education must understand these barriers and implement creative strategies for overcoming them. Common problems in health education and suggestions for addressing these problems are described here.

Language

There can be a failure to understand health promotion messages when language or symbols are misunderstood. A growing number of students and families do not speak English and/or are learning English as a second language. Therefore, it is important for teachers and school administrators to consider the impact that language may have in comprehension and ability to participate. Controversy surrounding bilingual education is unfounded. Bilingualism is not detrimental to cognitive development. Rather, bilingualism enhances thinking skills if the second language is learned in addition to, and with sustained development of, the native language (Hernandez, 1992).

Teachers must realize that families who speak English as a second language need written and verbal messages which are real, meaningful and understandable. Teachers can improve understanding by keeping form and content as simple as possible—modifying language by simplifying sentence structure and avoiding idioms and colloquialisms.

Language does not have to be a barrier, even when a family's primary language is other than English. Some schools offer English as a Second Language (ESL) classes for parents and this has proven a successful boost to family participation in schools. Additionally, take-home activities involving the family can provide opportunities for adult second-language learners to use English and participate in language development activities with their children.

Reading Level
Some printed materials may be too sophisticated or beyond the reading level of students and families. It is important that take-home activities, school-home notes, and other correspondence intended for families be written so that low-literacy families can understand them.

Inappropriate Messages
Messages that are not relevant to target group members will not be heard. Some messages may contain cultural bias reflecting beliefs, values, and/or practices which differ fundamentally from the family's belief and value system. It is especially useful to include family members in the planning of curricular materials and family involvement activities to ensure that these are applicable and acceptable.

Motivational Issues
Some families may fear that the primary motivation for a health promotion campaign is to control the subculture by robbing it of the specific practices that historically have defined it. To avoid this barrier, teachers and administrators must recognize and accept differences in a group's health beliefs and practices. Whenever possible, these differences should be incorporated in both class-

room instruction and in family involvement activities. For example, in the "Bright Smiles, Bright Futures" Oral Health Program, children were encouraged to discuss with their parents the myths or stories about what happens when they lose their teeth. Students, teachers and parents enjoyed this activity and commented that it was interesting to learn about the differences and similarities between cultures.

Relevance of Health Promotion

Families may feel that more pressing concerns, such as poverty, crime, unemployment and hunger, should be addressed prior to the health promotion campaign. To fully incorporate families in comprehensive school health programs, teachers and administrators should encourage input from families regarding health issues that are important to them. They should explain to families the linkage between various health topics and issues such as poverty, crime and unemployment.

Entropy

The tendency for group members to perceive themselves as powerless or helpless when confronted with enormous economic and sociocultural barriers, and to thus exhibit a lack of motivation to engage in self-improvement activities can be a barrier. Within the context of bettering the health of their children, families can often be motivated to promote a healthy environment in the home and assist in ensuring quality health education at school. Family involvement should aim to empower family members by providing them with suggestions, skills and knowledge to help their children and themselves reach higher levels of wellness. Families should be encouraged to participate actively in the health education of their children. As a result, families will not simply be given meaningless directions and advice. Instead, they will be involved in decision making and planning which directly affects both the educational experience of their children, and their level of participation at home.

Many of the barriers mentioned here occur mainly because of a lack of cultural awareness and/or sensitivity. One key to promoting family involvement in comprehensive school health education is the creation of an atmosphere of cultural awareness and acceptance.

Cultural Awareness and Sensitivity

Cultural sensitivity is a crucial component in the involvement of multiethnic parents in comprehensive school health education. Sensitivity should not only be reflected in the attitudes of the administration and teachers, but also in the health education curriculum. Cultural sensitivity implies that both cultural differences and similarities exist. Included in this belief is the refusal to assign to cultural differences such values as better or worse, more or less intelligent, or right or wrong. It is simply an acknowledgment that differences exist.

Problems in Defining Cultural Sensitivity
The term cultural sensitivity evokes a variety of different images, emotions and misconceptions. One misunderstanding of the term involves the belief that because persons are members of a particular cultural or ethnic group, they are implicitly culturally sensitive. This is not necessarily true. If people only interact within their own reference group, they may not be culturally sensitive. Insensitivity sometimes exists because there is no exposure to other ethnic groups. Another way of misinterpreting the term cultural sensitivity is believing that it refers to specific characteristics of the

members of a group such as sensitive, touchy, testy or fragile.

Many times, when discussing issues of cultural sensitivity, groups are divided into those who believe that sensitivity is needed and those who are perceived as insensitive. This establishes a culprit-versus-victim mentality, which sets up an automatic barrier between the two groups. Americans of European descent and others who make up the mainstream culture often feel defensive about the issue, and feel accused of fostering cultural insensitivity. The misunderstanding occurs when the concept of "culture" is limited to ethnic minority groups. Often members of the majority feel threatened or intimidated when discussing cultural sensitivity issues; many express a sense of distress at not belonging to a particular "culture."

We must recognize that *all* people have a culture, regardless of whether they are members of the majority or a minority group. Some members of majority populations will find it hard to identify or to get "in touch" with their roots. However difficult, it is important for people living in the United States to recognize that few of us (with the possible exception of Native Americans) are truly indigenous Americans. Most immigrated, sought political or religious asylum, or were brought in bondage to the United States; therefore, we have an ethnic origin that predates our American experience. Understanding this reality can help overcome the guilt or culprit-versus-victim mentality. Exercises that help families, teachers and administrators to identify the unique aspects of their own cultures can help to foster a better understanding about the role culture plays in daily life, and, particularly, in health behaviors.

In designing specific health education curricula and family involvement strategies we must learn that distinctive cultural and ethnic characteristics, customs, languages and needs make family living unique within each individual tradition. This diversity presents both a challenge and a potentially enriching experience to educators and parents alike. We must learn to value these cultural differences if we are to apply effective family involvement in health education.

Identifying Personal Biases and Beliefs

One of the most important steps in overcoming barriers to family involvement in the multiethnic classroom is for health educators to examine their own educational philosophies and cultural biases. Teachers may feel uncomfortable when dealing with people and issues that differ from their own experiences. These uneasy feelings often arise because of fear of the unknown. The sincere belief that one's own way of thinking or behaving is the correct or the best way may cause uncomfortable feelings to emerge when encountering others with different ways of thinking and behaving.

Recognizing our biases is really the first stage in becoming culturally aware. Furthermore, understanding these biases makes it easier to recognize the problems that children or families may have when interacting with people of other cultures. Ignoring cultural differences does not diminish them, rather, it increases resistance to creating acceptance and respect for others (AAHE, 1992). Once people become aware of their biases, they can go forward to create experiences that build comfort, acceptance and respect for persons of diverse cultures.

Another problem which can interfere with effective family involvement in a multicultural setting is stereotyping. We must avoid stereotypes when examining the health needs and concerns of ethnic minorities. Because of the way health statistics are presented, particular health problems are often attributed to certain ethnic groups. When discussing health problems affecting ethnic minorities, health educators should be careful to avoid particular phrases and statements, such as "you are more likely to become HIV infected if you are gay, Black or Hispanic." Health educators must emphasize, to both students and families, that it is behaviors and not characteristics of people that determine the prevalence of disease. Moreover, teachers must be wary of making assumptions about a particular family's health behavior based solely on their ethnic origin. For example, contrary to prevailing stereotypes, not all Mexican Americans use curanderos (folk healers).

Cultural awareness and sensitivity can certainly enhance the prospect of family involvement in health education. It is essential, however, to provide structure and mechanisms for families to participate. These mechanisms should be based on the fundamental principal that families should be partners in the education of their children.

Building Partnerships: A Plan for Action

"The partnership construct is based on the premise that collaborating partners have some common basis for action and a sense of mutuality that supports their joint ventures" (Swick, 1991). Teachers and families have a common goal: to foster the development and growth of their children while promoting their own growth as well. It is both a necessity and a challenge for families and schools to create a sense of shared commitment and mutuality so that efforts are productive and meaningful for all those involved (Swick, 1991).

The relationship between families and educators must move from the traditional role of parents as supporters and audience participants, to a collaborative, cooperative model of partnership. This model emphasizes sharing responsibility, information and power. Parents and educators complement each other in the education of children. Together they can provide a strong moral, emotional and scholastic base for children and convey to them a sense of stability and guidance. Family involvement is particularly important in health education, where family values, beliefs, individual cultures and expectations play critical roles in the understanding and assimilation of health information and in influencing health behavior. Parents, families, teachers and students must work toward the same goal.

Comprehensive, well-designed family education and family involvement programs can help provide the skills and knowledge critical to creating and sustaining a partnership model of health education. These programs must be designed, developed, implemented and evaluated with special attention to cultural awareness and sensitivity to better meet the needs of the variety of cultural and ethnic families and students that live in our communities (Amendolara, 1991). Families, administrators and teachers can take the following action-steps towards building these partnerships.

- Teachers and administrators can start building partnerships with families by promoting a philosophy of teamwork. This can be accomplished by making home visits, creating conferences and parent centers, telecommunication, classroom involvement, participatory decision making, parent and adult education programs, home learning activities, and family/school networking (Swick, 1991).

- Teachers can demonstrate their commitment to serving students and their families by developing, circulating and publicizing a specific statement of commitment. This may help establish credibility with populations that are traditionally underserved, or in many areas not served at all. The statement-of-intent of commitment should be printed in all languages and disseminated through foreign language newspapers, television and radio stations, and other media. Small language groups should not be ignored, since they may be the least likely to know about services.

A statement of commitment is strengthened by the position that an overall appreciation of American culture cannot be realized without an appreciation for its cultural diversity. We should regard differences and diversity as a societal strength, not a weakness. If this philosophy is explicitly stated in a message of commitment, it can help families of diverse cultural backgrounds feel accepted and welcome in the school and in the cooperative education of their children.

- Another important step in involving the family in comprehensive school health education is to actively seek their input. We can do this by conducting a "needs assessment" of their health concerns, and participation preferences. An assessment of family involvement needs does not necessarily have to be complex or time consuming. On the contrary, it can be quite straightforward and uncomplicated. For example, the principal of an elementary school began a major parent involvement effort several years ago by asking single parents how the school could help them. This straightforward and effective needs assessment provided parents with necessary support (e.g., childcare programs were set up, parenting education topics were offered). It also engendered a positive atmosphere between parents and school (Debusk and Leslie, 1991).

Teachers can improve their cultural awareness and sensitivity through a number of activities. To serve all students and families, the health education teacher needs to know:
- the names and geographic locations of families and their ethnic classification, including what specific cultures are represented

- the types of health problems the particular population group has, as well as health needs which may be more prevalent in certain groups
- their health beliefs and cultural tendencies surrounding disease, childbearing, family roles and relationships, and communication styles
- what situational variables must be taken into account, such as socioeconomic status, geographic location, resource availability, and residential stability

People interested in enhancing family involvement in a multicultural environment must consider the following (adapted from the AAHE Cultural Awareness and Sensitivity Training Project, 1992):

- There are many definitions of family. Definitions depend on individual experiences and ethnic backgrounds.
- Families should be viewed in their different forms. Be sure to include the specific family forms of all students represented in the school.
- Types of discipline and expressions of affection vary among families according to their ethnicity and culture.
- The importance of the family as a source of support and encouragement must be emphasized.
- Families may have different roles and expectations for children of different sexes. Cultural background may affect one's perception and experience of being male or female.
- In health matters, the active involvement of families should be particularly sought because families are the providers of primary life values.

Conclusion

Multiculturalism is much more than different dances, foods and games; it is an attitude which communicates to children, families and the community that diversity is desirable and acceptable. Multicultural health education is not just another issue, it is a specific approach to presenting instruction aimed at enhancing the health of the family and the community. It incorporates respect, understanding and celebration of various cultures. Teachers must promote discussion and awareness among students and their families regarding the cultural aspect of health issues and the identification of specific strengths, positive cultural models and practices for addressing some of the major health problems.

To realize community and family participation in health education we must address the specific sociocultural context and recognize the disadvantaged position of the United States' ethnic minorities. Family involvement in health education, from a multicultural standpoint, is a critical step in combining home and school health promotion. There is evidence that a multicultural perspective can promote positive health behaviors among both children and families, enhance child development and success, and ensure that minority children will have an equal opportunity to succeed.

References

Association for the Advance of Health Education. 1992. Training material. AAHE Cultural Awareness and Sensitivity Training Project.

Airhihenbuwa, C. O., and O. Pineiro. 1988. Cross-cultural health education: A pedagogical challenge. *Journal of School Health* 58 (6): 240-242.

Amendolara, L. P. 1991. The education community: Rewriting the script. *Momentum* 3:22-24.

Center for Education Statistics. 1987. *The Condition of Education.* Washington, DC.

Chavkin, N. F. 1989. A multicultural perspective on parent involvement: Implications for policy and practice. *Education* 109:276-285.

Chavkin, N. F., and D. L. Williams. 1985. *Executive summary of the final report: Parent involvement in education project.* Austin TX: Southwest Educational Development Laboratory.

Chavkin, N. F., and D. L. Williams, Jr. 1988. Critical issues in teacher training for parent involvement. *Education Horizons* 66:87-89.

Comer, J. P. 1986. Parent participation in schools. *Phi Delta Kappan* 67:442-446.

Debusk, S., and K. Leslie. 1991. How can we help? *Momentum: Journal of the National Catholic Education Association* (September): 25-28.

Elkin, D. 1991. The family and education in the postmodern world. *Momentum* 3:10.

Family Service America. 1987. *The state of families.* Milwaukee, WI: Family Service America.

Gold, R. S., M. Levy, C. Hide and M. E. Hernandez. 1992. *Bright smiles, bright futures: Final report of the Minority Oral Health Improvement Program.* College Park, MD: Laboratory for Health Promotion, Research and Development, University of Maryland.

Grant, C. A., and S. Millar. 1992. Research and multicultural education: Barriers, needs, and boundaries. In *Research and multicultural education: From the margins to the mainstream,* ed. Carl A. Grant. London: The Falmer Press.

Henderson, A. T., C. L. Marburger, and T. Ooms. 1986. *Beyond the bake sale: An educators' guide to working with parents.* Columbia, MD: National Committee for Citizens in Education.

Hernandez, H. 1992. The language minority student and multicultural education. In *Research and multicultural education: From the margins to the mainstream,* ed. Carl A. Grant. London: The Falmer Press.

Hodgkinson, H. L. 1985. *All one system: Demographics of education—kindergarten through graduate school.* Washington, DC: Institute for Educational Leadership.

Leitch, M. L., and S. S. Tangri. 1988. Barriers to home-school collaboration. *Educational Horizons* 66:70-74.

Louis Harris and Associates. 1987. *The Metropolitan Life survey of the American Teacher 1987: Strengthening links between home and school.* New York.

Montalvo, F. 1984. Making good schools from bad. In *Make something happen: Hispanic and urban high school reform.* Washington, DC: National Commission on Secondary Education for Hispanics.

Nader, P. R., J. F. Sallis, J. Rupp, C. Atkins, T. Patterson and I. Abramson. 1986. San Diego family health project: Reaching families through the schools. *Journal of School Health* 56 (6): 227-231.

Orlandi, M. A. 1986. Community-based substance abuse prevention: A multicultural perspective. *Journal of School Health* 56 (9): 394-401.

Orum, L. S. 1986. *The education of Hispanics: Status and implications.* Washington, DC: National Council of La Raza.

Pahnos, M. L. 1992. The continuing challenge of multicultural health education. *Journal of School Health* 62 (1): 24-26.

Rich, D. 1988. Bridging the parent gap in educational reform. *Educational Horizons* 66:90-92.

Swick, K. 1991. *Teacher-parent partnerships to enhance school success in early childhood education.* Washington, DC: National Education Association.

Underwood, C. 1986. *Schooling language minority youth.* Proceedings of the Linguistic Minority Project Conference, Berkeley, California, Vol. II, University of California Linguistic Minority Project, 102-108.

Wells, A. S. 1988. The parents' place: Right in the school. *New York Times Education Life* (3 January): 63-68.

Chapter 17

Community Partnerships in Comprehensive Health Education

Katherine-Kerry L. Bozza, MA

The children and youth in the United States today are growing up in an environment that encourages risk-taking behavior (Seffrin, 1990). Consequently, there is a growing realization that school health education programs must address the environmental factors which affect individual health behavior by increasing community involvement in school health promotion efforts. Many new and innovative health education methods have been developed based on current child developmental research. Models such as the PRECEDE model (Green and Iverson, 1982) suggest that the student be considered within the context of his/her family, community, and other social structures, rather than in isolation. However, there are still many school health promotion programs that do not fully consider the student within these contexts and that have subsequently had minimal results.

These health promotion activities have focused primarily on the predisposing and enabling factors an individual brings to a situation that affect whether or not a health-enhancing decision is made. They focus on behavior change as the responsibility solely of the individual. Research evaluating such activities suggests that these types of programs are successful with one time or occasional behavior, but do not seem to effectively change students' health-related behavior in the long term (Kirby, 1990). Currently, the school is still viewed as a primary change agent concerning youth health-related behavior. There is, however, a growing consensus among educators and health professionals that the school by itself cannot and should not be expected to succeed in changing long-term individual health behavior if the community environment in which an individual interacts continues to promote risk-taking behavior (Kirby, 1990; Green and Kreuter, 1990).

Changing health habits of youth or of any age group is already a very challenging task and becomes even more difficult if the desired behavior is not sufficiently reinforced. Society is comprised of individuals, groups and institutions that all give rise to and sustain health problems. Therefore, the prevention and promotion of health behavior should be a shared responsibility rather than the responsibility of the individual alone. It stands to reason that if health messages are consistently promoted throughout both the school and community, these messages will be much more effective. This chapter focuses on the integration of the school health program and the larger community to form a partnership that helps to create and maintain positive lifelong health habits.

The Need for a School/Community Partnership in Health Education

A school and community partnership in health education is necessary in order to reinforce and promote the health knowledge acquired in the classroom and to strengthen the social life and interchange within the community. Historically, schools have been considered an important mechanism for the promotion of the public's health primarily because of their ability to reach nearly 95 percent of all children and youth (Seffrin, 1990). Until 1984, health promotion activities involving the schools had traditionally been comprised of three major components: classroom school health education (instruction), school health services, and the school health environment (National Professional School Health Education Organizations, 1984). In 1987, research indicated that past school health promotion efforts that involved minimal outside intervention and focused primarily on the individual's responsibility for behavior change had only been able to sustain or slightly alter students' health behavior (Wilner, Walkley and O'Neil, 1978; Wallack and Winkleby, 1983). This resulted in a growing recognition of the importance of the environment in affecting a person's behavior and of the need to involve the surrounding school communities in school health promotion efforts. This recognition has been most evident in the recommendation by Allensworth and Kolbe in 1987 to include five additional components in comprehensive health education programs. One of these components is the involvement of the community in the school health promotion efforts (see Figure 1).

It is clear that the choices people make regarding their behavior "are intricately interwoven within the value systems, economics, and social fabric of their communities, families, social institutions, and ethnic and religious tenets" (Green, 1988). Thus, it has become increasingly important to involve the community in order to reinforce and strengthen the health promotion and educational efforts of the school. Research reviewing school health education programs that have linked the school and community and/or parents have shown significant differences in the acquisition of health knowledge and the practice of appropriate health behaviors

---

Figure 1
The Components of Comprehensive Health Education

1. School Health Instruction (Curriculum)

2. School Health Services

3. School Health Environment

4. Integrated Community and School Health Promotion Efforts

5. School Physical Education

6. School Food Service

7. School Counseling and Psychology Programs

8. School-Site Health Promotion Programs for Faculty and Staff

---

(Flay, 1985; Glynn, 1989; Vincent, Clearie and Schluchter, 1987). Such programs have been deemed successful primarily because "such community-based approaches typically combine interventions to enable families, peers, schools, media, and other relevant agencies within a community to address simultaneously a population behavior that influences health" (Kolbe, 1986).

Choices that individuals make regarding whether or not they will engage in risk-taking behavior are affected by numerous conditions within the community environment in which the individual interacts. Some of the environmental conditions that affect a person's behavior are of a personal nature. A person's age, income, level of education, feelings, values, beliefs and/or expectations all can either facilitate or inhibit behavior change. For example, as mentioned previously, past health education efforts tended to place all responsibility for health status upon the individual. Feelings of being solely responsible for one's own health status can lead to the development of low self-esteem and a sense of inadequacy. If disease results, the person feels low self-effi- cacy—that he or she does not have the capability to accomplish the task of prevention in order to maintain good health (Weitzer and Waller, 1990). Feelings of worth and self-efficacy are major influences on accomplishment of activities that individuals under- take. They determine the amount of effort and perseverance that the individual will bring to such activities. Changing the beliefs of the individual about her or his self-worth and self-efficacy can be an important part of changing behavior.

A person's individual relationships are also considered environ- mental conditions of a personal nature that can influence health- related behavior. Each person has a unique interpersonal and social environment comprised of parents, siblings, peers and other significant adults. Little dispute exists that people of any age can be greatly influenced by those who are important to them. The presence or absence of support that these people bring to a situa- tion can have a significant effect on a person's behavior. For example, a child who lives with parents who are excessive drinkers or drug addicts experiences a different home environment than a child whose parents abstain from drinking or taking drugs. Health habits are primarily learned from family, and, over time, become firmly established. These behavior patterns are later reinforced by interpersonal relationships within an individual's community.

Yet within an individual's community, health habits may often come to be performed automatically without awareness, and may never be examined or perceived as related to one's health status. However, what happens if an individual does become aware of a certain behavior and perceives it to be unhealthy? If the person makes a decision to stop performing the behavior, yet the commu- nity environment, which consists of family members and/or peers, does not perceive the behavior in the same manner and continues to support it, it is hard to imagine that the individual will success-fully stop performing the behavior. Community members such as parents, peers, teachers, school administrators and members of the law enforcement can all shape the immediate social environment in which young people live by supporting and promoting norms, attitudes and behaviors that decrease the likelihood of risk-taking behavior.

However, even if a school health promotion program instills positive self-esteem, increases a student's feelings of self-worth and self-efficacy, and creates more positive support from personal environmental conditions, the student may still be faced with other environmental conditions that prohibit positive health be-havior. Many of our youth and their families live below poverty level and do not have the money to access health services, let alone health insurance (Kirby, 1990). Also, the educational resources that help provide accurate and reliable health information to individuals, their families and their community are limited (Donatelle, Davis and Hoover, 1988). The youth of our nation experience inconsistent health messages and conflicting behavior standards and expectations that are shared by the members of a given community. Consequently, if an individual is faced with barriers, he or she will have a more difficult time engaging in positive health behavior if it is not supported and reinforced within the community.

When considering disease patterns and their associated lifestyles, it is essential to take into consideration the reinforcing factors present in the community environment in which a person lives when behavior change is desired. Even if the behavior change is adequately motivated and enabled, it will not persist unless it is reinforced. Therefore, it is reasonable to expect that school-based health programs will be more likely to succeed in influencing behavior when health-enhancing behaviors are promoted and reinforced throughout the community.

There are seven targets that any health education program should try to meet (Wilner, Walkley and O'Neil, 1978; Hunt and Martin, 1988; Donatelle, Davis and Hoover, 1988; Somers, 1976; Craig and Weiss, 1990; Sinacore, 1974):

1. When trying to promote behavior change, one must realize that people's behaviors already exist and are influenced by personal, social, cultural and physical factors in their environment.
2. Individuals must be motivated to change and must believe that they have the knowledge, skills and ability to do so.
3. Individuals must be made aware of the positive and negative forces in the environment that influence their health-related decisions.
4. If there is to be adherence and compliance to a change in a certain pattern in behavior, the change must be self-initiated and fit into the individual's mode of living.
5. Health education must promote the individual's sense of responsibility, self-esteem and level of self-efficacy.
6. The promotion of positive health behaviors must be made available, accessible and affordable.
7. Health education must be expanded into communities, schools, businesses, the media and the government, requiring everyone's participation to make it a comprehensive effort and not just an individual one.

All of these targets and recommendations recognize that the community is an integral adjunct to a child's health education, and that school and community health promotion efforts need to be strategically integrated. Health problems, especially those related to chronic diseases, cannot be reduced to individual behaviors as they were in old health education methods. These previous methods were aimed solely at the individual and assumed that people would be able to change even if the physical and social forces in the environment presented barriers to doing so. However, as we have seen, enabling, predisposing and reinforcing factors all act together to make behavior change either easy or difficult.

Therefore, it is essential for a school health education program to expand its individual health strategies to include the physical and social environment in its approaches as a means to "efficiently provide accurate health information; heighten community involvement; involve parents in their child's education; and develop a stable social network" (Iverson and Kolbe, 1983). Obviously the schools cannot, by themselves, influence the overall quality of the environment in which our nation's children and youth live. However, by involving parents and the community in a school health promotion program, we have the potential to:

- efficiently provide accurate health information
- bridge fragmented health services to form a more integrated system of health promotion
- increase accessibility and affordability of health services and information
- heighten parent and community involvement
- create a partnership in decision making with parents and the wider community across a range of issues which are of mutual concern
- increase parent/caretaker involvement in their children's education
- develop activities and programs that consider ethnic and cultural roots
- develop a network of community agencies that support the school and the cause of children's health.

Where to Begin

The challenge for each school and its community is to create their own unique partnership. It is important to take certain steps to ensure a cooperative working relationship. The following steps are offered as a recommendation of how to establish a partnership that will enhance the health of all children and their families in the school community. In order to establish a community partnership, educators must:

- Identify the community within which efforts will be concentrated.
- Develop a network of potential supporters.
- Create a health task force of school personnel and interested community parties.
- Working together, assess the varied needs of the school's youth and establish the norms, values and traditions of the community regarding health and proper health behavior.
- Establish priorities and goals, and develop integrated, collaborative programs and activities to meet them.
- Identify sources of necessary resources and become mobilized.
- Increase community awareness of health promotion efforts.

Identify the Community

The place to start when trying to involve the larger community in a project, is to first define the community. The success of a community mobilization effort will depend a great deal upon the type of community it is. A community can be large or small. It can be as simple as a few people who think of themselves as a group who share some common interests, concerns or activities. It can be a place where people share common public services (schools, parks, shopping centers, utilities), a residential area (town, neighborhoods, subdivision or block), or an institution (church, synagogue, neighborhood center, club, workplace, school). In the 1950s, schools generally served clientele who lived in close proximity to the school building. Each school was said to have its own "community" of interest. Since then, much has changed (DeFriese et al., 1990). Today the "school community" is difficult to define, primarily due to the increase in busing. This, in turn, has redefined the school community as being a collection of "neighborhoods." However one refers to the school community, each community is as special and unique as the people living within it.

American society includes a blend of some 250 million people. It contains communities which all differ in their accepted behaviors and practices, and are unique as to their demographic make-up, social and economic structure, leadership, culture, nationality, religion, health and well-being, values and communications. The population of the United States in 1988 was described as including "26.5 million African Americans, 1.4 million Hispanics, 3.5 million Asian/Pacific Islanders, and 1.4 million Native Americans (U.S. Department of Health and Human Services, 1986). The numbers have by now increased significantly, and, thus, the diversity of the communities within which we live has also increased. Evidence of a community's cultural diversity is apparent in the different languages, practices and beliefs that are intertwined within these groups. Although we use general labels like "African Americans," "Hispanics," etc., each of these groups are composed of people from various nationalities, compounding this tremendous diversity. These cultural differences ultimately have an impact on the health status of the population and on health programs that must be recognized for health promotion efforts to be successful.

Develop a Network of Supporters

The second thing to do is to identify existing health organizations and programs currently dealing with health issues concerning the youth population in the community. Many groups are already concerned about health education and prevention, and many other organizations have the potential to become involved.

Program advocates should create a list of these potential supporters and begin to develop a network of advocates for their cause who could make the difference between the success or failure of the partnership. Invite supporters to an awareness presentation and organize meetings to intrigue them with the need for health education among the community's youth. These preliminary meetings should be designed to establish a working relationship with the participants and to make them aware of the health problems of the youth. Once this relationship has been established, the interested parties should be invited to volunteer their efforts and become involved by representing their organization in a collaboration with the school health program on a school/community health task force.

Create a School/Community Health Task Force

A school/community health task force is necessary because members all have a common interest in health, and their different backgrounds will enhance the school's and the community's ability to see the need for implementation of a health event, something not always visible to an individual planner. The task force can serve multiple functions. It can help assess community needs and desires for education and survey current levels of health knowledge, attitudes, norms and behavior. It can also help to identify community resources and provide a mechanism for their utilization. Most important, task force members become advocates for the program and will be able to help represent the school/community health activities to the larger community.

Membership

The task force should include participants who are representative of community agencies, professional and religious organizations, voluntary health agencies, businesses, and community and parent groups. When health education programs are being planned, immigrant service agencies may also serve as an excellent resource. This is especially true when they are encouraged to get actively involved in the process, rather than just supply information to support the implementation of some predetermined program. Not only are such agencies conversant with the specific needs of a group in question, but they can also act as "conduits," linking health care agencies with their multicultural communities (Thompson and MacDonald, 1989). Most important, the task force should strive for diversity among its members and include interested community members who truly reflect the racial and ethnic diversity of the community. Efforts will be most effective if members from the community are actively involved in the planning and implementation of the task force programs, because people from within the community will add credibility and visibility to the health promotion activities. They have professional, social and family ties to the community and are usually familiar with local language preferences, beliefs and practices concerning risk-taking behavior.

Work on the task force is a voluntary effort made by people who work for organizations with their own regular program commitments. Requiring too much time and effort from task force members can be detrimental to the program. People will be more likely to volunteer for the task force if they know their specific duties, time commitment needed, location, project goals, training requirements and travel needs. If being a member of the health task force involves a number of different tasks, a brief job description should be sketched out for each task. Clear program goals will make it easier to locate volunteers and interest them in the project.

Sensitivity to Turf Issues

It is important to remember that specific organizations will volunteer their efforts because they are committed to a common cause but also to protect their own interests. Effective community task forces should not involve themselves too closely with specific projects or programs that existing community agencies, groups or organizations have already established. Organizations will withdraw their support if they feel that the task force activities duplicate, threaten or compete with their own existing programs. As mentioned previously, when identifying the community, it is very important to identify existing programs that could be incorporated into the plans and project goals. All other activities can then be created to fill in any gaps in health services and designed to incorporate existing services.

Maintaining Accountability

How well a community health task force can sustain members and live up to its objectives will greatly depend on the caliber of its coordinators. One of the first considerations of those responsible for organizing community involvement is to locate coordinators who can strengthen the interpersonal relations of all group members and maximize support for the group's objectives. In order to do this, it is important to identify the people who care most about doing something to stop the problems in their communities. Although outsiders, politicians and other professionals can be helpful, outside programs and experts come and go in communities, sometimes leaving little accomplished, and often end up creating skepticism among community residents about the possibility of change. Program planners must look for people who possess the skills needed by the group. Sometimes this will be someone who has excellent abilities in self-expression and persuasion—the kind of person who may seem like a natural leader.

At other times the group will need people who know how to organize citizens or obtain cooperation from the business community. These people may be less visible and may have no leadership skills other than their specific expertise. An outside expert cannot take the place of a local leader. Outside experts are not personally involved in the community, and including them in a project may prevent the development of local camaraderie. People are needed who are familiar with the general running of the school and its administration and who have a good understanding of and are full supporters of health education. They should also be able to communicate with the community in their language; have a good working knowledge of the community—including an awareness of the community's history, especially concerning past efforts to improve the health of youth; be acquainted with diverse people in the community; and have a willingness to work and go to meetings. Overall, they should be community people who have the reputation of getting things done, and they must be able to work effectively with many different kinds of individuals and groups.

Assess Needs of Youth and How These Are to Be Met

Together adults and youth set standards for acceptable behavior based on the culture and traditions of the community. These standards or norms exist in every community for every behavior. Perceptions of such community norms are believed to have a significant influence on health behavior. Therefore studying such community norms when planning a school and community partnership is extremely important. Every community is different, and each community/school partnership must be constructed and tailored to the specific needs of the community within which it is working.

Unfortunately, in the hurry to start work, many who engage in community-based efforts neglect this initial groundwork. To be effective, efforts to involve the community with a health program must be relevant to the health, social, economic, educational and cultural environment within the community and school. Since cultural differences and individual perceptions of community norms are believed to significantly influence individual behavior and the outcome in health status, health programs must be developed to address them. Assessment is particularly important in communities of ethnic minorities, especially when the people working to involve community members are not from these communities.

In culturally diverse communities, the potential for conveying irrelevant information is much greater, causing health promotion programs to be less effective. A needs assessment should be carried out to help prioritize goals and evaluate the existing health organizations and health programs available to the community. In order to do this, appropriate youth-serving organizations and other health-related organizations that have joined the health task force should be asked to offer assistance in the creation and implementation of the needs assessment and in the collection of the data. Schools can also assist in administering an anonymous questionnaire to their students to assess health knowledge, attitudes and risk-taking behavior.

There are several approaches that the task force members could take to perform a needs assessment in the community. They include but are not limited to:
- surveying community members at community forums and meetings
- case studies

- using social indicators
- service provider surveys
- key informant surveys
- target population surveys
- anonymous student questionnaires
- parent questionnaires during PTA meetings

Set Priorities and Goals
and Develop Programs and Activities

Once the youth population needs have been identified and the existing services and programs in the community for youth have been evaluated, it is important to set priorities and goals to meet the objectives for improving the health of the children and youth in the community. Greater priority should be given to those behaviors that are the most prevalent and the most amendable. Program planners must ask what needs of the children and youth are not being met and which of these the program will concentrate on during the upcoming school year. Given the array of information provided by the needs assessment, the task force can engage in consensus building to prioritize the important health problems and then identify the problems that could most easily be addressed and that the program could have the greatest impact on.

The partnership will need worthwhile projects to meet its objectives, projects that sustain the energy and enthusiasm of the participants and are relevant and meaningful to the social strengths of the community. Some techniques used in conjunction with a comprehensive health education program involving community members include:

- health screenings
- information hotlines
- lectures or workshops by community leaders and health professionals

- health fairs
- heart-healthy bake sales
- health clubs
- bowling leagues; jogging, or walking groups
- programs that offer job skills and careers in the health field
- health education programs
- heart-healthy cooking classes
- neighborhood programs such as safety watches or environmental clean-up days
- family or generational walks
- youth fitness programs in coordination with local health clubs
- family culture/history days in collaboration with local libraries and museums
- family and parenting courses related to health care and skills
- community health conferences or events such as the creation of nature walks and trails
- student/parent tobacco and drug prevention activities
- support groups

All of these approaches have one thing in common: they require a high degree of cooperation and collaboration among the schools, public health departments, hospitals, community health centers, youth-serving organizations, and, of course, the multi-cultural communities served by such organizations. Remember that the key to the partnership is to encourage and maintain consistent health information within the environment and to reinforce positive health behavior.

Identify Community Resources
Once planners and the task force have decided upon the issues on which to concentrate efforts, they must ask what resources are needed to achieve these objectives and goals. The objectives deter-

mine the resources. The efficient implementation of a speaking program, for instance, requires a backup speaker to avoid disappointment if the primary speaker cannot attend a scheduled event. Similarly, displaying posters requires community support. It may, for example, require a supply of letterhead stationary for formal requests to the owners of property where posters will be located. A systematic effort to list all needed resources during the planning phase tends to prevent problems arising during implementation if a small but crucial item has been overlooked. It is important to utilize all possible resources and to do so it is important to examine all programs existing in the community. Knowing what health organizations, services, programs and resources already exist in the community and which would be appropriate to bring into the partnership program via a special quest speaker and/or an already-established event will save a lot of time and energy.

Many resources may be needed in order to reach the goals; these can be physical as well as less tangible. For example, a comprehensive school program often requires an investment of time and work by volunteers. It also may require expert knowledge of specialized topics or the cooperation of people and organizations to implement/enforce the information taught in the school through the health curriculum. All of these resources must be identified and secured to carry out a successful community- and school-based prevention program. Many of them are called "in-kind" services. A business, for instance, may not be able to provide actual dollars, but it may be able to print a brochure if allowed to include its logo. Alternatively, a business may be able to lend a public relations expert or an accountant for one day a month. In-kind donations are often as valuable as actual dollars.

The final part of this planning step is to decide where the resources will come from. Many feel that integrating the school health program within the community and with established community health programs would be a substantial burden, especially to school health personnel. This does not necessarily need to be the case. Partnership responsibilities may be divided and assigned to community members and health organizations that have been identified as already dealing with particular youth health issues and that can extend their programs and services into the school environment. Many of the resources needed can be obtained through contributions from the community/school health task force members, such as volunteer labor and access to facilities for special events. Others may be more difficult to obtain. This should not be discouraging, however, because the community is a valuable reservoir of resources. Resources can be found at the local level, among the school staff, the parents, religious organizations, throughout the local community, and even among the students themselves.

Local museums and libraries often have staff who are experienced in the education system and already have a special responsibility for liaison with schools. Many local voluntary organizations of a charitable kind can provide materials, links and visiting speakers in connection with the topic area of cultural diversity in communities and health promotion. People from local charitable organizations who may have particular cultural experiences and insights could be valuable contributors to the program. Local businesses can be asked to sponsor parts of the program. Places of business such as banks, grocery stores, retail shops, children's stores, and restaurants can be utilized to display various artwork and projects, such as paintings, posters, essays, and/or pictures of children involved in the activities. Local media, sororities and fraternities, nursing and medical students, small business associations, churches and religious organizations, and youth-serving organizations that are not health related should all be reviewed to see if they can contribute to the program. Thus, community involvement can open up new resources and make the local community feel that it is appreciated and that its diversity of cultures is fully recognized.

Increase Community Awareness

Once the programs and agendas of the partnership have been established, it is important and most beneficial for a partnership to increase the awareness of its activities within the larger community. Such a partnership will make some wonderful things happen and sharing these things with the community is very appropriate and beneficial for all involved. Utilize all media relationships that the organizations, community members and school have already established. Send press releases to all radio stations, newspapers, magazines and television stations that include upcoming health-related activities and programs, as well as cite the number of children who are being positively affected as a result of the partnership. Make sure names, addresses, and telephone numbers are included so that the activities and programs can be contacted for more information. The more the word gets out to the community, the more credibility the program will have and the more positive publicity it will receive.

Promoting Multiculturalism Throughout

An important aspect of promoting health in schools and in the community is acknowledging the integral role played by individuals' cultures and ethnic backgrounds. As we have seen, it is important to identify the various cultures and ethnicities of the school population and the communities that the students are from in order to understand the environmental conditions that students face in regard to promoting positive health behavior. It is important for a community partnership to include members from the community who represent the specific cultural and ethnic makeup of the members. It is important to recognize the existence of different cultural groups who maintain some separate structures, traditions and norms, yet also hold some structures, norms and health practices in common with all other groups of society. Members of different cultural groups may be faced with the same fragmentation of health care services or may be presented with the same amount of incorrect and inconsistent health information.

For partnership programs to be successful, they need to be tailored to the needs and norms of the designated community. They must support the social structure and ethnic makeup of the community population. Activities such as heritage days, family fun days, or ethnic heart-healthy bake sales or potluck community suppers that support positive health behavior and offer supportive environmental conditions for student interaction will be beneficial. Also, incorporating such organizations as media, businesses, sororities and fraternities, will heighten awareness of the program and strengthen its ties to all aspects of the community. Only when activities truly represent the community and its unique characteristics, will the students be able to apply and integrate health information into their lives.

Conclusion

Due to the many environmental variables and conditions that individuals face, education agencies at every level must work closely and cooperatively with corresponding health agencies and community members on an ongoing basis in order to promote consistent, positive health messages. A partnership will help to create new linkages and networks among community residents, health care providers and services, and will serve to reconnect the community itself. Involving parents, siblings and community agencies in school health promotion programs demonstrates to students that health education, while taught in the school, is applicable to their "real lives." Community, school and family involvement reinforces positive social norms regarding health and provides additional motivation for making health-enhancing decisions.

School and community health programs "need to be strategically integrated to attain community input in the design of school health programs; to acquire community support for the implementation and maintenance of school health programs; and to achieve health-related behavioral impact among students" (Iverson and Kolbe, 1983). As summarized in the 1988 report The Forgotten Half, "Efforts to produce success in school without complementary efforts in families and communities are unlikely to make a substantial difference for young people." School health programs should be viewed and structured as collaborative efforts between schools, parents, community and religious leaders, civic organizations, physicians, politicians, psychologists, social workers and the media as a way of building and reinforcing a sense of community by rallying the diverse elements of an individual's environment to address a common concern.

References

Allensworth, D., and L. Kolbe. 1987. The comprehensive school health program: Exploring an expanded concept. *Journal of School Health* 57 (10): 409-412.

Craig, K. D., and S. M. Weiss. 1990. *Health enhancement, disease prevention, and early intervention.* New York: Springer Publishing Co.

DeFriese, G. H., C. L. Crossland, B. MacPhail-Wilcox and J. G. Sowers. 1990. Implementing comprehensive school health programs: Prospects for change in American schools. *Journal of School Health* 60 (4): 182-187.

Donatelle, R. J., L. G. Davis and C. F. Hoover. 1988. *Access to health.* Englewood Cliffs, NJ: Prentice Hall.

Flay, B. R. 1985. Psychological approaches to smoking prevention: A review of findings. *Health Psychology* 4:449-488.

The forgotten half: Pathways to success for America's youth and young families. 1988. Final report, Youth and America's Future: William T. Grant Foundation Commission on Work, Family and Citizenship.

Glynn, T. 1989. Essential elements of school-based smoking prevention programs. *Journal of School Health* 59 (5): 181-187.

Green, L. W. 1988. Bridging the gap between community health and school health. *American Journal of Public Health* 78:1149.

Green, L. W., and D. C. Iverson. 1982. School health education. *Annual Review of Public Health* 3: 321-338.

Green, L. W., and M. W. Kreuter. 1990. Health promotion as a public health strategy for the 1990s. *Annual Review of Public Health* 11:319-334.

Hunt, S. M., and C. J. Martin. 1988. Health related behavioral change: A test of a new model. *Psychology and Health* 2:209-230.

Iverson, D. C., and L. J. Kolbe. 1983. Evaluation of the national disease prevention and health promotion strategy: Establishing a role for the schools. *Journal of School Health* 53 (5): 294-302.

Kirby, D. 1990. Comprehensive school health and the larger community: Issues and a possible scenario. *Journal of School Health* 60 (4): 170-177.

Kolbe, L. J. 1986. Preventing drug abuse in the United States: Integrating the efforts of schools, communities, and science. *Journal of School Health* 56 (9): 357.

National Professional School Health Education Organizations. 1984. Comprehensive school health education: A definition. *Journal of School Health* 54 (8): 312-315.

Seffrin, J. 1990. The comprehensive school health curriculum: Closing the gap between state-of-the-art and state-of-the-practice. *Journal of School Health* 60 (4): 151-155.

Sinacore, J. S. 1974. *Health: A quality of life.* New York: Macmillan.

Somers, A. R. 1976. *Promoting health: Consumer education and national policy.* Aspen Systems Corporation.

Thompson, P. R., and J. L. MacDonald. 1989. Multicultural health education: responding to a challenge. *Health Promotion* (Fall): 8-11.

U.S. Department of Health and Human Services. 1986. Health Status of the Disadvantaged Chart Book. Washington, DC.

Vincent, M. L., A. F. Clearie and M. D. Schluchter. 1987. Reducing adolescent pregnancy through school and community-based education. *Journal of the American Medical Association* 257 (24): 3382-3386.

Wallack, L., and M. Winkleby. 1983. Primary prevention: A new look at basic concepts. *Social Science and Medicine* 25 (8): 923-930.

Weitzer, M. H., and P. R. Waller. 1990. Predisposing factors for health promotive behaviors on Whites, Hispanics and Black blue collar workers. *Family and Community Health* 13 (1): 23-33.

William T. Grant Foundation. 1988. *The forgotten half: Pathways to success for America's youth and young families.* Final report, youth and America's future. William T. Grant Foundation Commission on Work, Family and Citizenship.

Wilner, D. M., R. P. Walkley and E. J. O'Neil. 1978. *Introduction to public health.* New York: Macmillan.

Appendix

Ethnic and Demographic Profiles

This appendix presents ethnic and demographic data relevant to planning and implementing multicultural health education.

Figure 1 presents enrollment in public school data and compares 1986 and 1990 enrollment for 27 states where African-American, Hispanic, Native-American and Asian-American students in elementary and secondary public schools exceed 20 percent of the student population. In the majority of the cases the ethnic population has grown from 1986 to 1990.

Figure 2 presents an ethnic profile of early elementary school children (ages 5 to 8).

Figure 3 offers projections of the Hispanic population of the United States through the year 2080. Hispanics are the fastest growing ethnic group in the United States.

Figure 4 presents data on the number of persons who speak a language other than English at home.

Taken together, the data in these figures help make a strong case for the importance of a multicultural approach to health education.

Figure 1

Enrollment in Public Elementary and Secondary Schools, by Race or Ethnicity and State: Fall 1986 and Fall 1990

State	Percent distribution, fall 1986						Percent distribution, fall 1990					
	Total	White[1]	Black[1]	Hispanic	Asian or Pacific Islander	American Indian/ Alaskan Native	Total	White[1]	Black[1]	Hispanic	Asian or Pacific Islander	American Indian/ Alaskan Native
United States	100.0	70.4	16.1	9.9	2.8	0.9	—	—	—	—	—	—
Alabama	100.0	62.0	37.0	0.1	0.4	0.5	100.0	62.8	35.7	0.2	0.5	0.7
Alaska	100.0	65.7	4.3	1.7	3.3	25.1	100.0	67.5	4.4	2.1	3.7	22.3
Arizona	100.0	62.2	4.0	26.4	1.3	6.1	100.0	63.1	4.1	24.5	1.5	6.8
Arkansas	100.0	74.7	24.2	0.4	0.6	0.2	100.0	74.5	24.2	0.5	0.6	0.2
California	100.0	53.7	9.0	27.5	9.1	0.7	100.0	45.6	8.6	34.4	10.6	0.8
Colorado	100.0	78.7	4.5	13.7	2.0	1.0	100.0	75.3	5.2	16.3	2.3	0.9
Connecticut	100.0	77.2	12.1	8.9	1.5	0.2	100.0	74.9	12.7	10.1	2.2	0.2
Delaware	100.0	68.3	27.7	2.5	1.4	0.2	100.0	68.0	27.4	2.9	1.6	0.1
District of Columbia	100.0	4.0	91.1	3.9	0.9	0.1	100.0	3.9	89.8	5.2	1.1	(2)

[1]Excludes persons of Hispanic origin.   [2]Less than 0.05 percent.   —Data not available.
Source: U.S. Department of Education, National Center for Education Statistics. 1992. *Digest of Educational Statistics.* Washington, DC.

Figure 1 (continued)
Enrollment in Public Elementary and Secondary Schools, by Race or Ethnicity and State: Fall 1986 and Fall 1990

State	Percent distribution, fall 1986						Percent distribution, fall 1990					
	Total	White[1]	Black[1]	Hispanic	Asian or Pacific Islander	American Indian/ Alaskan Native	Total	White[1]	Black[1]	Hispanic	Asian or Pacific Islander	American Indian/ Alaskan Native
United States	100.0	70.4	16.1	9.9	2.8	0.9	—	—	—	—	—	—
Florida	100.0	65.4	23.7	9.5	1.2	0.2	100.0	61.9	24.0	12.4	1.5	0.2
Georgia	100.0	60.7	37.9	0.6	0.8	(²)	—	—	—	—	—	—
Hawaii	100.0	23.5	2.3	2.2	71.7	0.3	100.0	22.6	2.4	2.7	72.0	0.3
Illinois	100.0	69.8	18.7	9.2	2.3	0.1	100.0	65.7	21.6	9.8	2.7	0.1
Louisiana	100.0	56.5	41.3	0.8	1.1	0.3	100.0	53.2	44.4	1.0	1.1	0.4
Maryland	100.0	59.7	35.3	1.7	3.1	0.2	100.0	61.1	32.9	2.3	3.5	0.2
Michigan	100.0	76.4	19.8	1.8	1.2	0.8	100.0	78.3	17.2	2.2	1.2	1.0
Mississippi	100.0	43.9	55.5	0.1	0.4	0.1	100.0	48.3	50.7	0.2	0.4	0.4
Nevada	100.0	77.4	9.6	7.5	3.2	2.3	100.0	74.2	9.0	11.3	3.5	2.0

[1]Excludes persons of Hispanic origin.   ²Less than 0.05 percent.   —Data not available.

Source: U.S. Department of Education, National Center for Education Statistics. 1992. *Digest of Educational Statistics.* Washington, DC.

385

Figure 1 (continued)
Enrollment in Public Elementary and Secondary Schools, by Race or Ethnicity and State: Fall 1986 and Fall 1990

State	Percent distribution, fall 1986						Percent distribution, fall 1990					
	Total	White¹	Black¹	Hispanic	Asian or Pacific Islander	American Indian/ Alaskan Native	Total	White¹	Black¹	Hispanic	Asian or Pacific Islander	American Indian/ Alaskan Native
United States	100.0	70.4	16.1	9.9	2.8	0.9	—	—	—	—	—	—
New Jersey	100.0	69.1	17.4	10.7	2.7	0.1	100.0	65.2	18.6	11.7	4.4	0.1
New Mexico	100.0	43.1	2.3	45.1	0.8	8.7	100.0	42.2	2.3	44.8	0.8	9.9
New York	100.0	68.4	16.5	12.3	2.7	0.2	100.0	66.2	16.6	12.9	4.1	0.3
North Carolina	100.0	68.4	28.9	0.4	0.6	1.7	100.0	66.5	30.3	0.8	0.9	1.6
Oklahoma	100.0	79.0	7.8	1.6	1.0	10.6	100.0	74.2	9.9	2.7	1.1	12.1
South Carolina	100.0	54.6	44.5	0.2	0.6	0.1	100.0	57.8	41.1	0.4	0.6	0.1
Tennessee	100.0	76.5	22.6	0.2	0.6	(²)	100.0	76.3	22.5	0.3	0.8	0.1
Texas	100.0	51.0	14.4	32.5	2.0	0.2	100.0	49.6	14.4	33.8	2.0	0.2
Virginia	100.0	72.6	23.7	1.0	2.6	0.1	—	—	—	—	—	—

¹Excludes persons of Hispanic origin.   ²Less than 0.05 percent.   —Data not available.

Source: U.S. Department of Education, National Center for Education Statistics. 1992. *Digest of Educational Statistics.* Washington, DC.

Figure 2
The Ethnic Profile of School Children
in the United States

The following population totals are for children ages 5 to 8 years old.

White males	18,861,469
White females	17,848,317
African-American males	3,715,062
African-American females	3,629,436
American Indian, Eskimo or Aleut males	270,865
American Indian, Eskimo or Aleut females	259,950
Asian or Pacific Islander males	826,706
Asian or Pacific Islander females	729,146
Males of Hispanic origin	2,982,337
Females of Hispanic origin	2,814,569
Other race males	1,380,144
Other race females	1,307,132

Source: U.S. Department of Commerce. 1992. *1990 Census of Population and Housing: United States Summary*. (1990 Summary Tape File 1C). Washington, DC.

Figure 3
Projections of the Hispanic Population of the United States: 1983–2080

Highlights

- The Hispanic population may double within 30 years and triple in 60.
- The White Non-Hispanic population may peak in size by 2020 and then steadily decrease.
- Even without international migration, the Spanish-origin population may grow more quickly than would most other major population groups with immigration.
- The Hispanic population shows tremendous growth.
- All Spanish-origin age groups would experience substantial future growth; in fact, all would double in size within 50 years.
- The Spanish-origin population is growing about three times as quickly as is the total population and will continue to do so through 2080.

Projections of the Population, by Age, Race and Spanish Origin: 1982–2080
Numbers in thousands
Total (5–17 years):

Spanish Origin:
1995: 5555
2000: 6207
2030: 8458

Black:
1995: 7871
2000: 8321
2030: 8917

White Non-Hispanic:
1995: 33,712
2000: 33,830
2030: 28,778

Other Races:
1995: 1705
2000: 1775
2030: 2551

In summary, all group populations will be increasing in the next forty years, except White Non-Hispanics.

Source: U.S. Bureau of the Census. 1986. Gregory Spencer, Current Population Reports, Series p. 25, No. 995, Projections of the Hispanic Population: 1983 to 2080. Washington, DC.

The Multicultural Challenge in Health Education

Figure 4
Persons Who Speak a Language
Other Than English at Home

Persons 5–17 Years
Total: 6,322,934
Percent who do not speak English "very well":   37.8%

Persons 18 and Older
Total: 25,522,045
Percent who do not speak English "very well":   45.4%

Source: U.S. Department of Commerce. 1992. 1990 Census of Population and Housing: Summary Social, Economic and Housing Characteristics, (1990 CPH-S-1). Washington, DC.

Contributors

Veronica M. Acosta-Deprez, PhD, CHES, is presently a faculty member of Health Promotion at the Department of Health and Human Performance at Auburn University, Auburn, Alabama. Her professional interests include multicultural health education; class, race and gender issues in health care and health education; school health; community health education; and the integration of instructional technology into the field of health. She has had experience in several areas of nursing and has worked as a health educator and researcher in the Philippines. She has also contributed articles and made presentations in the field of multicultural health education.

Collins O. Airhihenbuwa, PhD, MPH, is an associate professor of health education and an affiliate faculty member of the Department of African/African American Studies at the Pennsylvania State University. His research focuses on the relationship between cultural identity and health behaviors among Africans and African Americans. He has developed a culturally sensitive programmatic model for planning, implementing and evaluating health promotion programs among Africans and African Americans. Based on his international health and cultural health research, he has conducted many seminars and workshops at the local, national and international levels using his model as a framework. He is a consultant to several national and international organizations.

Loren B. Bensley, Jr., EdD, CHES, has been a secondary school teacher of health education and a university professor for the past 33 years. Presently he is a professor of health education and health science at Central Michigan University where he teaches curriculum and methods classes in health education. He has been an advocate for comprehensive school health education and has served the profession in many leadership roles including president of the Michigan and the American School Health Association. His interests in multicultural diversity evolved from experiences which included teaching, consulting and doing research in six European countries. He believes that a practical approach to multicultural health education includes understanding and appreciating diverse groups, being knowledgeable about specific health problems of multiethnic communities, and the application of appropriate methodology.

Michael E. Bird, MSW, MPH, is the associate director of the Office of Preventive Health Programs for the Albuquerque Area Indian Health Service (IHS). In this role he has supervisory responsibilities for eight preventive programs serving 27 tribes in New Mexico, Colorado and Texas. He has extensive experience in prevention program development and implementation with American Indian populations. He has been involved in the development of culturally relevant approaches that build on the strengths and positive cultural values inherent in indigenous cultures. He is the past president of the New Mexico Public Health Association.

Katherine-Kerry L. Bozza, MA, is the curriculum development coordinator for the comprehensive K-6 health promotion program "Know Your Body." She directs the development of the curriculum and is involved in its dissemination and implementation nationally as well as internationally. In this capacity she also has had the opportunity to train teachers, youth service organizations and health coordinators in comprehensive school health promotion. She currently serves on a committee called "TRAC" that is dedicated to the enhancement of healthy teenage relationships and communications in her home town of Greenwich, Connecticut.

Karen L. Butt, EdD, is currently an assistant professor at California State University, Los Angeles. She has written numerous articles and done extensive research in the area of multiculturalism in health education, physical education and general education. She received her EdD in 1989 from the University of North Carolina at Greensboro.

Antonio Casas, MA, is a doctoral candidate in counseling psychology at the University of California, Santa Barbara. His research and clinical interests focus on acculturation and in particular how counselors adapt to assist clients with acculturation issues during the counseling process. In addition, he is interested in the relationship between the acculturation process and specific symptomatology that clients may bring into the counseling process.

J. Manuel Casas, PhD, received his PhD in Counseling Psychology from Stanford University and is currently a professor in the Counseling, Clinical and School Psychology Program at the University of California, Santa Barbara. He has worked extensively with Hispanics and other racial/ethnic minority groups and is presently devoting much of his time to identifying specific sociocultural variables and institutional interventions that contribute significantly to the success and/or failure of ethnic minorities in social, educational and corporate settings. He has published widely in the area of cross-cultural counseling and education. Along with Joseph Ponterotto he is the co-author of the *Handbook of Racial/Ethnic Minority Counseling Research.* He has served on numerous editorial boards including the *Counseling Psychologist,* the *Journal of Multicultural Counseling and Development* and the *Journal of Hispanic Behavioral Sciences.* As president of JMC and Associates he serves as a consultant to various governmental agencies, organizations and corporations that are interested in working more effectively to meet the diverse needs of individuals from racial/ethnic minority groups.

Lillian Vega Castaneda, EdD, is associate professor of education at California State University, San Marcos, where she coordinates the (Bilingual) Crosscultural Language and Academic Development (B/CLAD) teacher preparation program. Her primary research areas include the identification and description of exemplary educational practices for culturally, linguistically and ethnically diverse students, bilingual and cross-cultural education, and the nature of language and literacy in mainstream, multiple-language and bilingual contexts. She was the associate study director of A Descriptive Study of Significant Features of Exemplary Special Alternative Instructional Programs, a national study commissioned by the U.S. Department of Education. Currently, she is conducting applied research in the area of whole language and literacy instruction in Spanish and multiple-language instructional contexts. She holds a doctorate in Teaching, Curriculum and Learning Environments from Harvard University.

Linda R. Comfort, RN, MPH, is the Program Director/Clinical Supervisor for the School Health Program Private/Parochial Schools, for the City of Boston, Department of Health and Hospitals, Division of Public Health. She directs the health services and health education programs to forty private/

parochial schools in the city of Boston. She also coordinates maternal and child health services in East Boston and Charlestown. She began her career with a focus on women's health and has worked in public health for over a decade.

Sally M. Davis, PhD, CHES, has worked with multiethnic communities in school health programs for the past twenty years. She is the principal investigator and project director for two National Institutes of Health primary prevention programs with Navajo and Pueblo schoolchildren that have developed culturally appropriate curricula and related educational materials. As an assistant professor and director of the Division of School and Preventive Health in the Department of Pediatrics at the University of New Mexico School of Medicine, she developed and teaches an experiential module in school and preventive health for pediatric residents and graduate students. She is the founder and editor of *Health Wise—A Bulletin for School Health,* now in its fifteenth year of publication, and heads the pediatric department's Office of Creative Endeavors, which supports faculty and staff in developing innovations in patient care, teaching, child advocacy and research.

Charlene A. Day, MPA, CHES, is the president of C.A.D. Associates, a consulting firm providing program planning, management and evaluation expertise to health education programs. As a Certified Health Education Specialist, she has worked extensively in the field of alcohol and substance use prevention and directed a national HIV/AIDS education and prevention program targeting college students. Over the past two years she has traveled around the country providing cultural awareness and sensitivity training for health educators in consultation with the Association for the Advancement of Health Education. She has recently completed the coursework required for a doctorate degree in health education and is currently working on her dissertation in the area of cultural sensitivity.

Deborah A. Fortune, PhD, CHES, is an assistant professor of health education at the University of North Carolina at Charlotte. She has provided training in cultural diversity in school health education, instructor training in comprehensive school health (*Growing Healthy* curriculum and *Teenage Health Teaching Modules*), and HIV/AIDS education for African Americans. Her research interests include minority health issues, HIV/AIDS among minority populations, child and adolescent health risk behaviors, and multicultural issues in school health education.

Ira E. Harrison, PhD, MPH, is an associate professor in the Department of Anthropology, University of Tennessee, Knoxville. He has conducted research on junior-senior high school dropouts, church desegregation, and health-seeking behavior among African Americans in neighborhood health centers and the Migratory Farm Labor System. His current research includes community HIV/AIDS awareness education.

Maria E. Hernandez, MA, received her BA in Spanish, BS in physiology and MA in health education from the University of Maryland, College Park. She is currently a PhD student in the Department of Health Education at the University of Maryland, with major areas of study in health promotion in special populations and public health. She has extensive experience in the formative and process evaluation of health education materials for people of color, including multimedia interventions. She is currently Deputy Project Director at Marco for the development of an interactive video disc on cancer prevention for Hispanic women. Previously, she was employed as a faculty research assistant in the Laboratory for Health Promotion Research and Development at the University of Maryland, where her research efforts focused on Hispanic health issues, including development of curriculum materials, translation and back-translation of health-related materials, and evaluation of a national minority oral health improvement program. She has played a leading role in planning and conducting focus groups on a variety of topics with Hispanic populations and has served as a consultant on several projects dealing with Hispanic health issues, including the process evaluation of a compact disc interactive program for Hispanic women.

Leonard Jack, Jr., PhD, is an adjunct assistant professor with the Department of Community Health and Preventive Medicine at Morehouse School of Medicine in Atlanta, Georgia. He has served as Director of Community Health Intervention within the Health Promotion Resource Center, Morehouse School of Medicine. Other teaching experience includes the Pennsylvania State University and Howard University. He has authored numerous presentations at noted conferences addressing HIV/AIDS education, substance use prevention, cancer prevention and control, community health education, multicultural approaches to disease prevention, and stress and general well-being among African-American youth.

Mark Jager, MS, is an assistant professor of health education at New Mexico State University, Las Cruces. He is currently a doctoral candidate at the University of New Mexico. His background includes hospital-based health promotion and administration.

William M. Kane, PhD, CHES, is associate professor of health education at the University of New Mexico in Albuquerque. He is a former public school teacher and coordinator of health education and an author of health education textbooks. He has served as executive director of two national health organizations, the Association for the Advancement of Health Education and the American College of Preventive Medicine, and has been active in the establishment of many national health education initiatives. He is the author of *Step by Step to Comprehensive School Health: The Program Planning Guide* (ETR Associates, 1993).

Ana Consuelo Matiella, MA, is Editor/Staff Writer for ETR Associates in Santa Cruz, California. Ms. Matiella specializes in multicultural education and the development of low-literacy health education materials for diverse populations. She is the author of *Positively Different: Creating a Bias-Free Environment for Young Children*; *The Multicultural Caterpillar*; *We Are a Family*; *La Familia* and *Cultural Pride*. Ms. Matiella has edited numerous books, fotonovellas and curricula for ETR Associates, including *Teaching Family Life in the Multicultural Classroom* and the *Latino Family Life Education Curriculum*.

Jeanne M. Mongillo, RNC, MPH, is a School Health Consultant for the City of Boston, Department of Health and Hospitals, Division of Public Health. She provides health services and health education programs for students, faculty and staff for six inner-city parochial schools in the city of Boston. She began her career working in pediatric acute care and then focused her efforts in community-based public health work. She has had extensive experience in worksite wellness programs, community-based childbirth education programs and school-based health education programs.

Marie J. Montrose is Director of Patient Relations at Interfaith Medical Center in New York City. A native of Haiti, she is particularly concerned with the accessibility of health education and services for immigrants and minorities. She lectures extensively on consumer rights in health care. Ms. Montrose resides in Brooklyn, where she volunteers as an HIV/AIDS and pregnancy prevention counselor for newly immigrated teenagers.

Maria Natera, EdD, an educator, researcher, trainer and management consultant, is founder and president of Natera and Associates. She has four years experience as a public school teacher, eighteen years as a site and district office administrator, and has served as an adjunct professor at CSU Sacramento, the Universities of Santa Clara and San Francisco, and National University. Her work in cross-cultural communications and as a consultant in organizational development in the workforce has earned her recognition among educators, government agencies, nonprofits and the private sector. She conceptualized the workshop Beyond the Golden Rule based on the belief that cultural diversity is an advantage if it is understood, esteemed and well managed. Beyond the Golden Rule teaches that cultural diversity is not simply to be tolerated but to be encouraged, supported and nurtured. Despite her busy schedule, she finds time to pursue her second love—filmmaking—and has received several commendations for her creative use of training technology.

Markella L. Pahnos, PhD, is currently an associate professor and director of school health programs at Springfield College in Massachusetts. She has written numerous articles and done extensive research in the area of multicultural education. She teaches a graduate course in multicultural health education and includes course work in multicultural issues throughout the undergraduate and graduate curricula. She received her PhD in health education in 1984 from the University of Pittsburgh.

Rima E. Rudd, ScD, a member of the faculty and the Director of Educational Programs in the Department of Health and Social Behavior, Harvard School of Public Health, teaches courses on public health program planning and health education strategies, and is engaged in a variety of departmental and research projects. She began her career as a high school teacher in New York City and subsequently focused on community-based health education programs in her work with schools, hospitals, unions, professional organizations and community groups. Her work in participatory materials development is one aspect of her interest in a new pedagogy for public health.

Anthony R. Sancho, PhD, is currently the associate director of the Desegregation Assistance Center at the Southwest Regional Laboratory (SWRL) in Los Alamitos, California. Prior to that, he was the director of the Hispanic Health Education Center at the Lab. For the last twenty years, he has been involved in the development of curriculum and training programs for teachers and administrators working with language minority students. He has delivered technical assistance to school districts and educational institutions throughout the country, and has been involved in the evaluation of programs addressing the needs of limited English proficient youngsters. When he directed the Hispanic Health Education Center, he developed a national reputation expressing his concerns about risk behaviors that affect the learning of Latino youth in American public schools. He has also been involved in the development of multicultural training materials for teachers working with African-American, Asian, Hispanic and Native American students.

Lisa Shames, PhD, received her bachelor of science degree in biological sciences from California Polytechnic State University, San Luis Obispo, in 1986. She received her master's of Public Health in epidemiology and biostatistics from San Diego State University in 1989, followed by a doctorate in health education at the University of New Mexico in 1993. She has recently been awarded an NIH post-doctoral fellowship at the University of Southern California School of Medicine where she will be studying the effects of diet and hormones with respect to reproductive neoplastic diseases.

Iris M. Tropp, MA, works as a school health consultant. She formerly directed comprehensive school health programs for the National Education Association's Health Information Network. Prior to joining the Health Information Network, she coordinated a New York City AIDS prevention project for in-school adolescents through Columbia University's HIV Center. She has taught health at all levels and has written a variety of health education materials. Her primary focus is the integration of school health education with other social and community services. She holds a master's degree in Health Advocacy from Sarah Lawrence College.

Nina Wallerstein, DrPH, is an assistant professor in the Department of Family and Community Medicine, School of Medicine, University of New Mexico. For the last twenty years, she has adapted the empowerment education and transformational philosophy of Paulo Freire to health education, community organizing, adult and youth education, and public health. She is director of the Adolescent Social Action Program (ASAP). Her interests include the role of powerlessness in disease, and empowerment in health enhancement, community participation and the development of healthier communities.

Linda M. Zani, RN, is a public health nurse and works in two parochial schools as a School Health Consultant for the City of Boston, Department of Health and Hospitals, Division of Public Health. She also provides home health visits for perinatal services. She began her nursing career providing acute pediatric care and has had extensive experience in management and health care delivery. She offers services to the Boys and Girls Clubs and youth programs in Boston, serves on numerous community task forces addressing a wide range of public health issues, and designs and implements community-based health education programs.

Index

The Multicultural Challenge in Health Education

The Multicultural Challenge in Health Education

learning styles and, 284–286
motivating students, 113–114
organizing learning experiences, 142
power dynamics, 167–168
protection-motivation method, 171
sheltered instruction, 237–238
strategies for family involvement,
340–341
Total Quality Management (TQM),
overview, 263–264

V
Vietnamese. *See* Asian Americans
violence prevention, 194–196

Y
youth, minority. *See* minority youth